Raising the Bar

The Definitive Guide to Pull-up Bar Calisthenics

By Al Kavadlo, CSCS

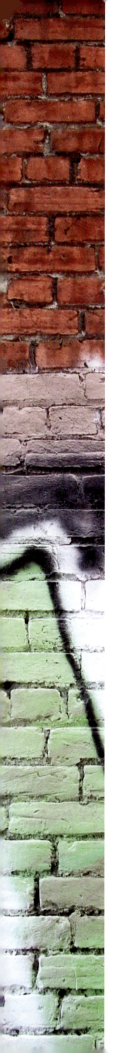
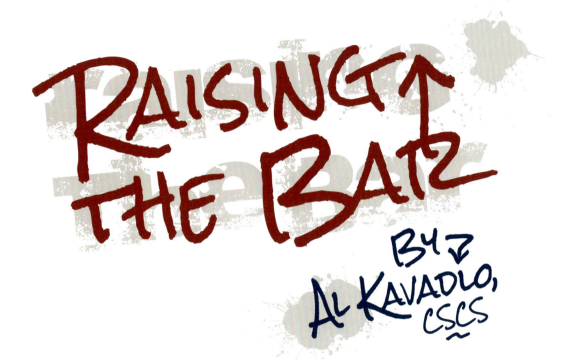

RAISING THE BAR
By Al Kavadlo, CSCS

Copyright 2012, Al Kavadlo
A Dragon Door Publications, Inc production
All rights under International and Pan-American Copyright conventions.
Published in the United States by: Dragon Door Publications, Inc
5 East County Rd B, #3 • Little Canada, MN 55117
Tel: (651) 487-2180 • Fax: (651) 487-3954
Credit card orders: 1-800-899-5111 • Email: support@dragondoor.com • Website: www.dragondoor.com

ISBN 10: 0-938045-45-8   ISBN 13: 978-0-938045-45-8

This edition first published in May, 2012
Printed in China

No part of this book may be reproduced in any form or by any means without the prior written consent of the Publisher, excepting brief quotes used in reviews.

Book design and cover by Derek Brigham • www.dbrigham.com • (763) 208-3069 • bigd@dbrigham.com

Photography by Colleen Leung • www.ColleenLeung.com
Cover photo: Colleen Leung • Back cover photo: Tamar Kaye • About the author photo: Darius Vick

Illustration on page 154 by William Gadol

Models: Christian Barnes, Christina Camerlingo, Kiki Flynn, Rodney "Redd" Harrison, Meng He, Rob Hollander, Keith Horan, Jennylynn Jankesh, Al Kavadlo, Danny Kavadlo, Colleen Leung, Kristin Leung, Chinyere Sam, Rick Seedman, Lord Vital, Synkwan "Syn" Yam. Additional models provided by Barstarzz (www.Barstarzz.com): Shaun "Swiss" Bryant, Eduard Checo, Jason "Sick With It" Fernandez, John Hendricks, Jose "Vertical" Jimenez, Juan Rosario.

Additional photos: Al Kavadlo, Danny Kavadlo, Tamar Kaye, Abdiel Munoz, Billy Lee Silva

DISCLAIMER: The author and publisher of this material are not responsible in any manner whatsoever for any injury that may occur through following the instructions contained in this material. The activities, physical and otherwise, described herein for informational purposes only, may be too strenuous or dangerous for some people and the reader(s) should consult a physician before engaging in them.

– Table of Contents –

Introduction – The Truth Hurts	1
Chapter 1 – Pull-up or Shut-up	5
Chapter 2 – Oh Dip!	29
Chapter 3 – Hard Core Training	47
Chapter 4 – Advanced Pull-ups	65
Chapter 5 – Enter The Muscle-up	83
Chapter 6 – Handstands and Shoulder Health	109
Chapter 7 – Lever or Leave 'er	135
Chapter 8 – Zen and The One Arm Pull-up	155
Chapter 9 – The Bar Brotherhood	167
Chapter 10 – Beyond the Bar	177
Appendix: Sample Routines	187
Acknowledgements	191
About The Author	193

Raising the Bar

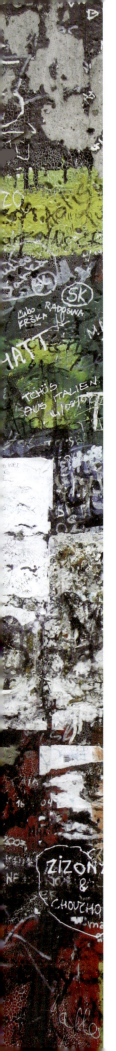
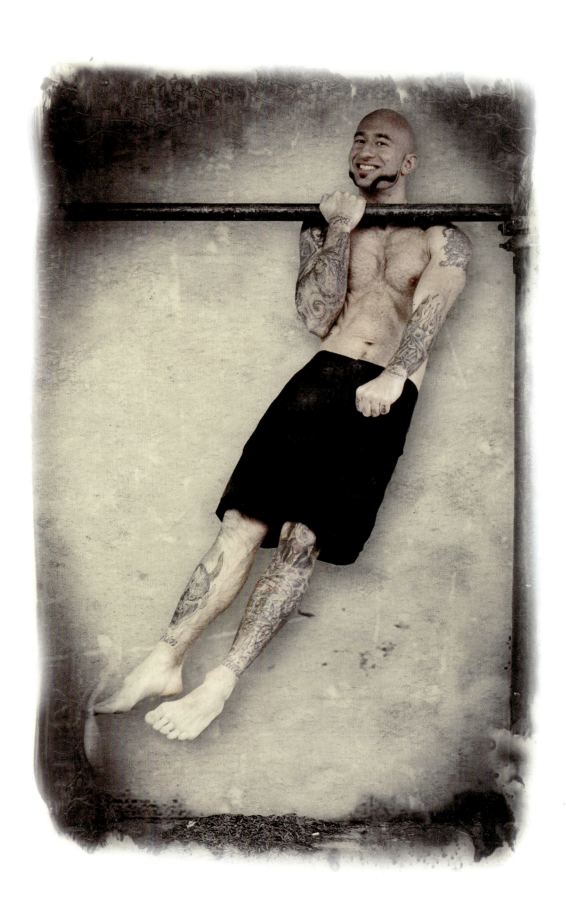

FOREWORD
By Paul "Coach" Wade

A heavily muscled urban athlete lines up under the high bar and looks up at it grimly. He's oblivious to his surroundings; the cars streaming past, the kids playing and shouting all around, the noise of the city. All he sees is that bar—he knows it's the key to the extra muscle and power he needs to build.

A lean, tattooed convict queues up in the yard to work out on the rusty pull-up unit—he may only be able to use it twice this week, and he's got to get his workout done fast and efficiently if he wants to stay on top of his game.

An elite gymnast arrives at the gym for her early morning session. After a brief warm-up, she heads to her second home—the horizontal bars. The true training is about to begin.

Some icy rain begins to spit as a tough, grizzled marine hops up to grip the iron chinning bar left outside the barracks. Like endless generations of warriors and soldiers before him, he's mastering his bodyweight. Pull-ups, pull-ups, and more pull-ups for this wily vet.

What do all these fearsome athletes have in common? They're using that damn bar! And with pretty good reason, too: the simple horizontal bar is the most important piece of strength and conditioning equipment there is—bar none. ('Scuze the pun.) My mentor, Joe Hartigen—one of the great "unsung heroes" of physical culture—always used to say that a horizontal bar was the *only* essential piece of training equipment. He believed that you could replace the barbell with floor calisthenics (*one-arm push-ups, bridges, one-leg squats,* etc.) but there was no way to replace the value of a horizontal bar. You've just gotta work that bar!

Joe was right. Bar training is *indispensable* for strength athletes. Even if you are a hardcore lifter, you still need to train with a horizontal bar to unlock your maximum potential. Why? Physics. I learnt at least one fact back in school—on earth, gravity only ever pulls things *downwards*. (I didn't stick around to find out why; something to do with apples, I think.) This means that when you lift weights, or perform floor calisthenics, you are only ever moving things *up*. Deadlifts, curls, push-ups, squats, cleans—you're lifting things up, right? As great as these exercises may be, if you are only ever lifting up, you are building your body in an asymmetrical way. You need to pull *down* as well—and this requires a fixed bar.

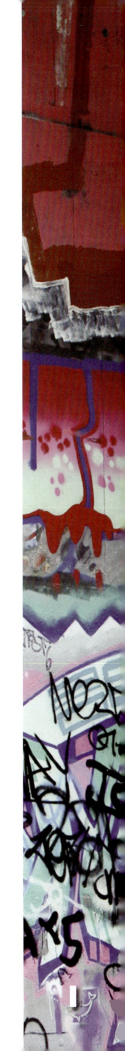

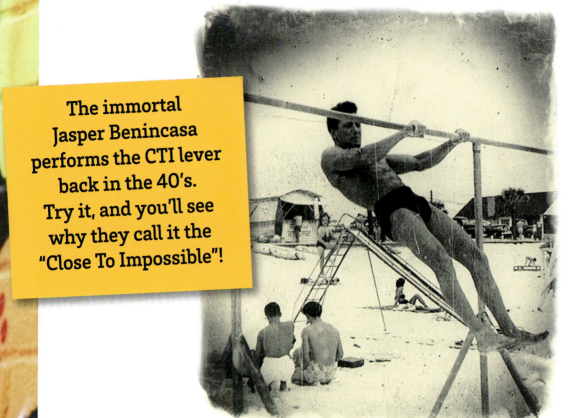

The immortal Jasper Benincasa performs the CTI lever back in the 40's. Try it, and you'll see why they call it the "Close To Impossible"!

Working with the fixed bar unleashes *ferocious* functional strength. A lot of coaches talk about "functional" strength, and give different definitions. For me, functional strength is *the ability to move your own body through space*. Other types of strength may be useful, but they all proceed from functional strength. This is the strength you need to escape an emergency—climb a wall, ramp over a fence, etc. Bar athletics is the ultimate "tester" of functional strength. It's totally unforgiving. I know a lot of big, fat power-lifters who can pull huge amounts of iron in the gym. But can they do a *muscle-up*? A *front lever*? Five *rollovers*? No way!

Sadly, very few athletes devote enough time and energy to the bar. When they do, they see bar training as "pull-ups". This is a damn shame. Just as an expert lifter can use a barbell to perform a wide number of exercises, so a bar athlete can perform many different types of productive technique. Apart from the extensive family of pull-up techniques (*archer pull-ups*, anyone?), you can also perform an equally huge range of dips, presses, grip and ab exercises. The bar is also a great place for incredible total-body moves like *muscle-ups* and *skinning the cat*.

RAISING THE BAR

Why is the bar so misunderstood and underused? Part of the problem is that there has never been a definitive high-quality training manual on working with the bar. If you think about it, this is nuts. There are literally *thousands* of books dedicated to machine work, barbells, dumbbells and kettlebells. But have you ever seen a comprehensive encyclopedia devoted specifically to bar training? Nope, me neither!

...Until now.

This here book is something very special. It's likely the most important book on strength and conditioning to be published in the last fifty years. That's a big claim, but I stand by it. Not only is it of historical importance as the only book I've ever seen that's dedicated to bar athletics—the "missing link" of strength training—but it's also a phenomenal conditioning resource in its own right. In this book you'll learn all the techniques you need to succeed; you'll find out how to dominate different types of bar setups; you'll discover how to combine and balance your bar moves with other advanced training techniques, like handstand push-ups; and, just as crucial, you'll be taught to forge all these new skills into a routine of laser-like efficiency.

What makes this book even more exciting is it's author—"supertrainer" Al Kavadlo. Al is a modern master of bar athletics. His skills on the bar are beyond belief, and his ability to think "outside the box" in training and coaching are rapidly becoming a thing of legend. I could go on and on about Al, but I won't. I'll just say that after twenty years learning calisthenics behind bars, there's only one man alive I go to when I have questions on bodyweight training. His name is Al Kavadlo.

If you only ever get your hands on one training manual in your life, make it this one. Buy it, read it, use it. This book has the power to transform you into the *ultimate* bar athlete.

Heck, I'm excited for ya! There's a horizontal bar near you, right? In a gym, a park, a sports field?

...Then what're you waiting for, kid?

Paul Wade

Paul Wade 2012

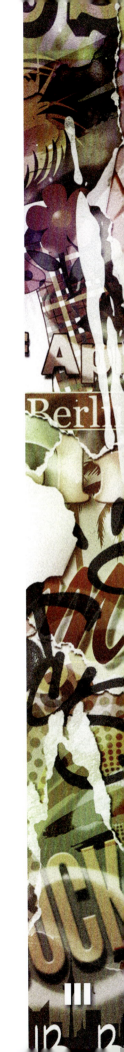

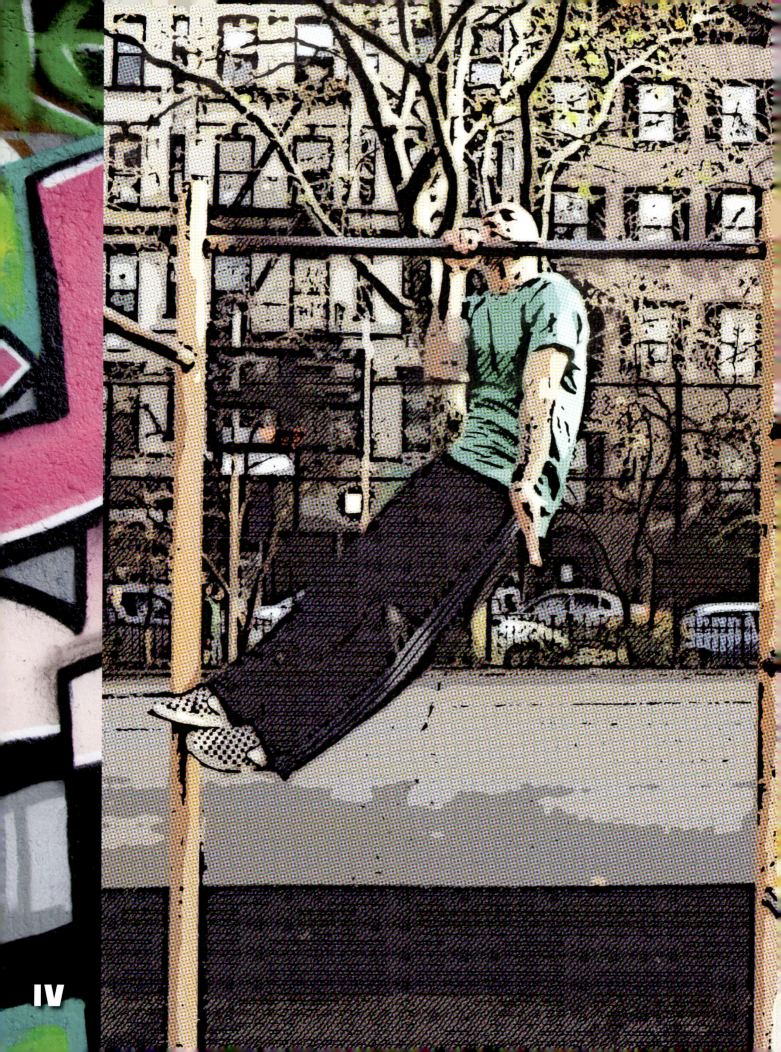

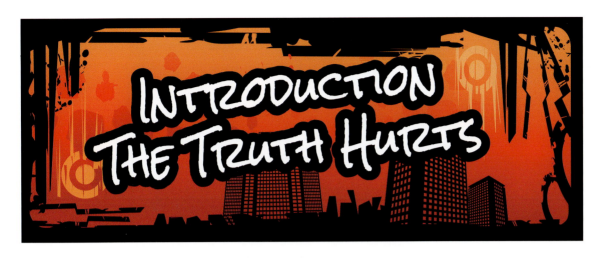
Introduction: The Truth Hurts

"I want the truth!"
"You can't handle the truth!"
–from *"A Few Good Men"*

When I tell people they don't need weights or a gym membership to get in the best shape of their lives, you would think they'd be relieved. They don't have to spend their hard earned money or even leave their home to get fit - this should come as good news! Usually the opposite happens, though. People are often disappointed by my advice, even skeptical. It seems too simple to be true. After all, if you could get fit with no gym membership, no machines and even no weights, then how come it hasn't happened yet?

Well that's the thing, fitness doesn't just happen - you have to make it happen! A gym membership can't make it happen and neither can buying a treadmill or purchasing a shiny new set of weights. Accepting that none of those things really matter means accepting that it is all up to you, which can be a very difficult thing to do. Accepting responsibility means that if you are out of shape, it's your own damn fault. But that's the beauty of it, too - you don't need anything outside of yourself to get fit - you have all the power. Once you are truly committed to health and fitness, the only limitations are the ones you impose on yourself. On the path toward greatness, the only thing that matters is that you consistently dedicate yourself to improving. You have to be willing to do the work. Muster up some gumption and don't give up when the going gets rough. Once you start doing that, the rest will take care of itself.

The truth is that while getting fit is simple, it's not easy - and it's never going to be. There are going to be moments where it hurts. There will be times when you want to stop — you might even want to cry. But if you push through those moments, you will wind up not only with a body that is physically stronger, but a mind with strength beyond what you ever knew before.

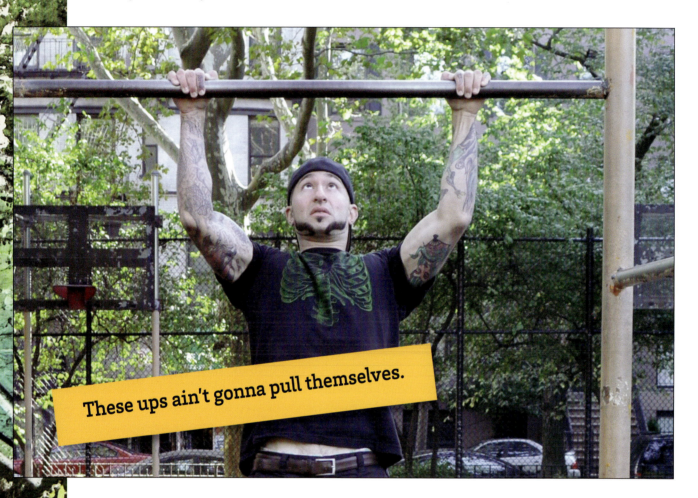

These ups ain't gonna pull themselves.

Nothin' But the Bar

You honestly don't need any equipment to get fit, but if you are looking for a workout apparatus that can do it all, you need look no further than the basic pull-up bar. It's far and away the simplest and most versatile piece of equipment in the world of fitness.

Though the possibilities are limitless in the world of bar training, there are basically just three types of exercises that you can do: pull-ups, dips and hanging leg raises. Everything else is more or less just a variation (or a combination) of those fundamental moves. That's right, just three basic moves, but endless variations to keep you challenged for a lifetime.

What about legs?

It's a bit of a cliché that guys who train pull-ups have chicken legs. Check out any of the amazing videos of bar athletes on YouTube and you're bound to see comments criticizing them for not having well developed legs. While you can't take the average YouTube comment too seriously, it's true that any athlete (or regular person for that matter) will benefit greatly from training their lower body. Believe me, I'm all about working your legs. I can deadlift twice my body weight, do twenty pistol squats on each leg and I've run a Marathon - but this book is about the bar, and the bar is for training your upper body.

One more thing, even though push-ups are one of my favorite exercises, I'm not going to get into them in this book. Push-ups deserve a whole other book of their own! Though I will discuss a couple of non-bar exercises here, the program in this book is designed around bar training. Feel free to work push-ups into your routine, but you can honestly do fine without them if you do everything in this book.

I'm glad we got all of that out of the way early on.

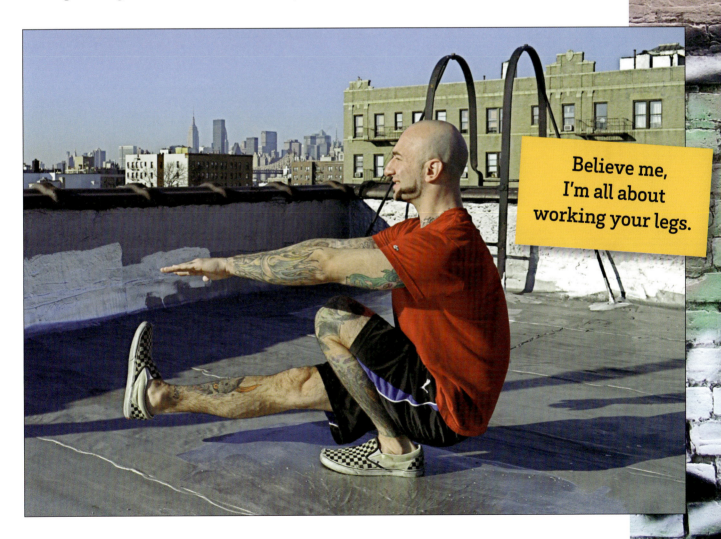

Believe me, I'm all about working your legs.

Level Up

I'm about to give you all you'll need to know to build a strong, powerful upper body and a chiseled set of washboard abs. If you follow my plan, you are guaranteed to feel better, perform better and of course, look better. Of course, YOU still have to do the work.

So the only question that remains is, "Are you ready to take things to the next level?"

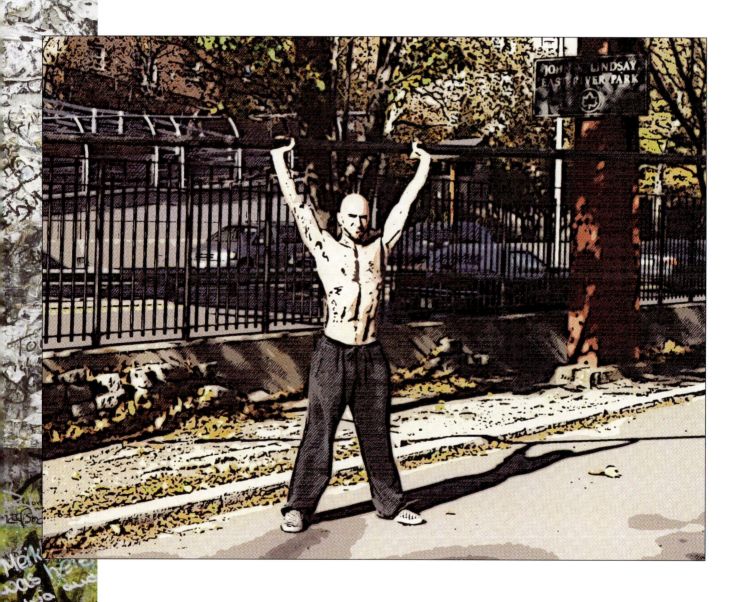

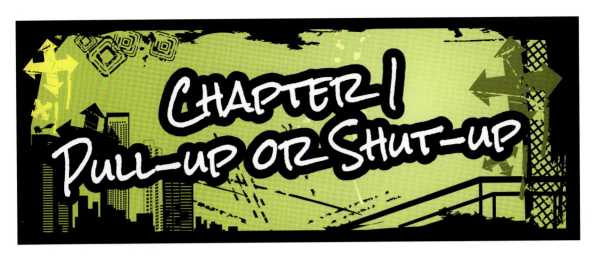

Chapter 1
Pull-up or Shut-up

> "A wise man speaks because he has something to say, a fool speaks because he has to say something."
> –Ancient Proverb

The first piece of fitness equipment I ever owned was a pull-up bar. I got it when I was thirteen years old and installed it in the doorway of my bedroom. Since I was so light, I was actually able to do a couple of chin-ups right away. (Chin-up is the technical name for a pull-up done with an underhand grip.)

Though the trusted pull-up has always had a place in my workout regimen, over the years I've spent a lot of time seeking out new innovations and experimenting with different training modalities in an attempt to progress my fitness. My desire to find the perfect workout led me to try barbells, dumbbells, kettlebells, weight machines, cable machines, stability balls, medicine balls, sandbags, jump ropes, and anything else I could find. Surely there had to be a machine or some kind of wobbly device that could get me in peak physical condition. But alas, I've come full circle in my training, leaving behind all the weights, machines and other "innovations" in favor of training my upper body with nothing but the bar and my own bodyweight.

The pull-up is my all-time number one favorite exercise simply because it's the purest way to measure or train pound-for-pound strength. Pull-ups are the great equalizer, putting the little guys on a level playing field with the big boys. They are the source from which all bar calisthenics are borne.

RAISING THE BAR

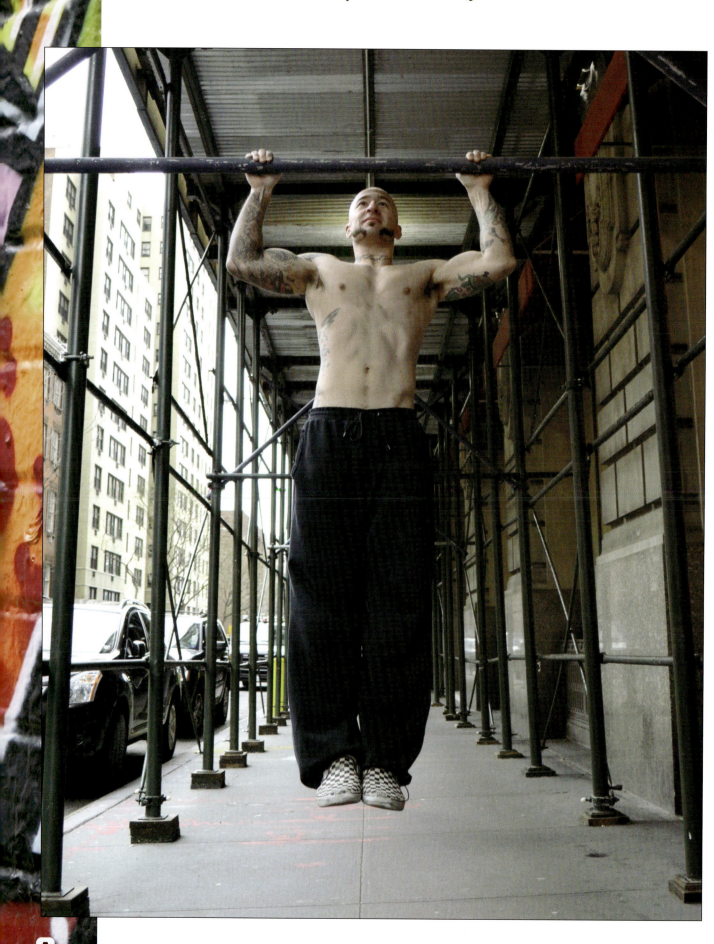

Raising the Bar

No matter how strong you think you are, pull-ups can be humbling. The bar can be your best friend or your worst enemy - that's up to you. It's better to be quiet and let your actions speak for themselves. Remember that no matter how far you go on your journey, there is always uncharted land ahead. Nobody is the best at everything and the world of bar training is bigger than you might think. Ignore those who may offer advice but fail to back it up in their performance. You can watch all the calisthenics videos in the world, but until you get under the bar and really start pulling your weight around, you'll never understand what it's all about.

Ladies and Gentlemen

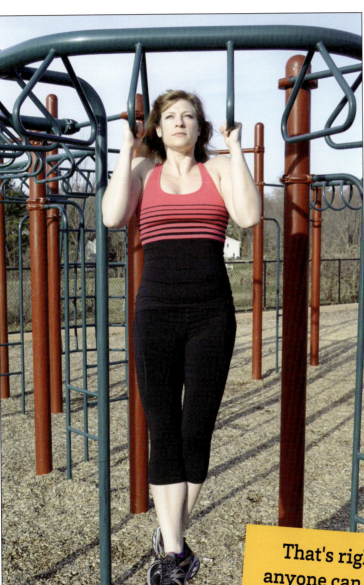

Females can be especially intimidated by the bar, but let me assure you, women can do pull-ups! It might be a little more work for the ladies, but it is within the potential of every able-bodied woman to perform a pull-up.

Some women may be concerned that pull-up bar training will make them too muscular. I can't tell you how many times I have heard this myth perpetrated. Being afraid that pull-ups will make you too muscular is like being afraid that reading books will make you too smart; it's really just an excuse for those who aren't willing to make the effort. Sadly, this misguided notion prevents many females from achieving their potential.

That's right, ladies – anyone can do pull-ups!

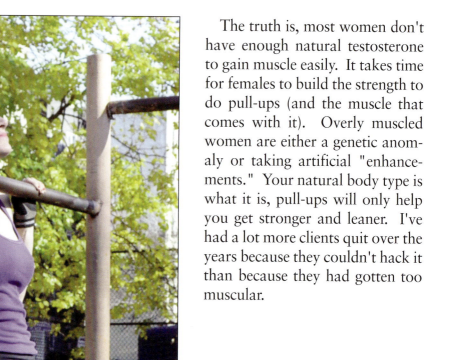

The truth is, most women don't have enough natural testosterone to gain muscle easily. It takes time for females to build the strength to do pull-ups (and the muscle that comes with it). Overly muscled women are either a genetic anomaly or taking artificial "enhancements." Your natural body type is what it is, pull-ups will only help you get stronger and leaner. I've had a lot more clients quit over the years because they couldn't hack it than because they had gotten too muscular.

Regardless of gender, if you aren't strong enough to do a pull-up yet, fear not - a pull-up bar is still the best piece of fitness equipment you could ever own. As you work your way up to your first pull-up, you can use the bar to help you get there.

There are three primary exercises that you can do on an overhead bar as a precursor to a pull-up: flex hangs, negatives and dead hangs.

RAISING THE BAR

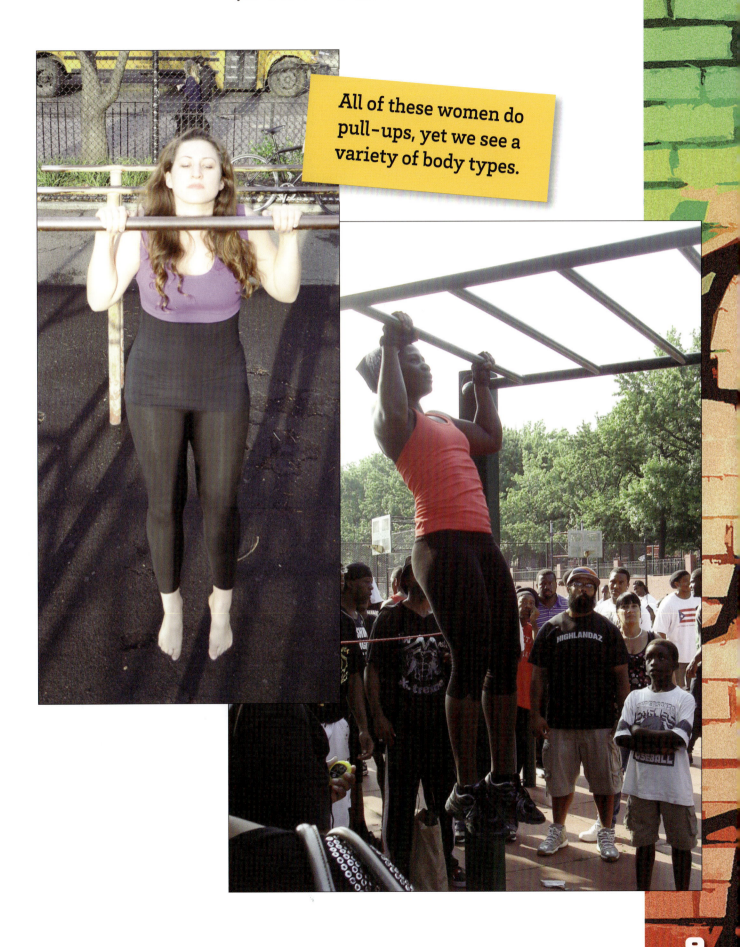

All of these women do pull-ups, yet we see a variety of body types.

Flex Appeal

A flex hang involves holding yourself at the top of a pull-up with your chin over the bar. It is best to start using an underhand (chin-up) grip. Use a low bar, a bench or a partner to help you get in position and then simply try to stay up. Use your arms, your back, your chest and even your abs to help maintain this position. Think about squeezing every muscle in your entire body. This concept of creating total body tension is essential for many of the exercises that are performed on the bar. The flex hang is a wonderful way to begin developing that ability. If you can hold this position for even a second on your initial attempt, you are off to a good start.

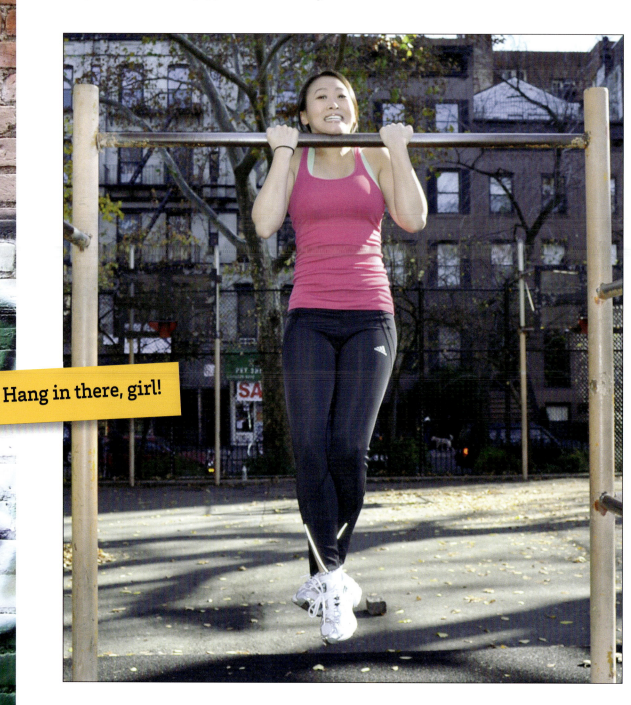

Hang in there, girl!

Negative Creep

Once you can hold the flex hang for several seconds, you're ready to start working on negative pull-ups, which just means lowering yourself down slowly from the top position. In the beginning, it might be very difficult to perform a controlled negative, but with time you will be able to make your negative last for ten seconds or longer. Though you want to make the rep last for as long as you can, don't try to move in slow-motion, instead think of lowering yourself at a normal speed and freezing for half of a second every inch of the way down. This will help you stay in control. Imagine a photographer is trying to take a series of photos and you need to be still during each shot.

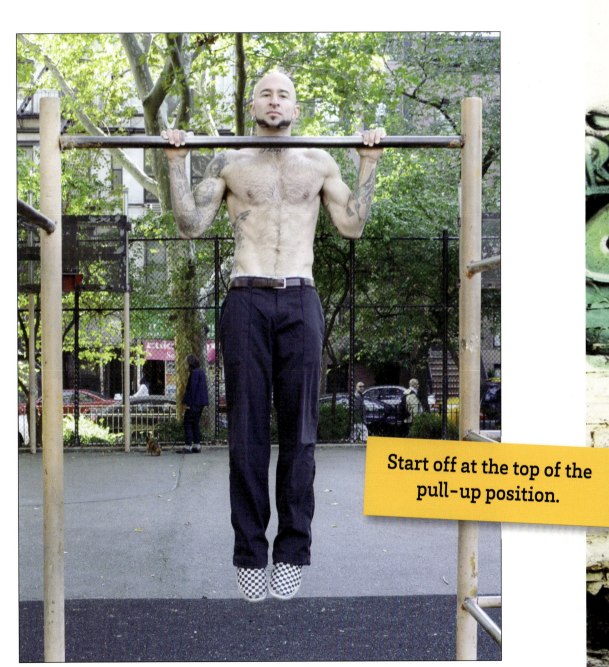

Start off at the top of the pull-up position.

RAISING THE BAR

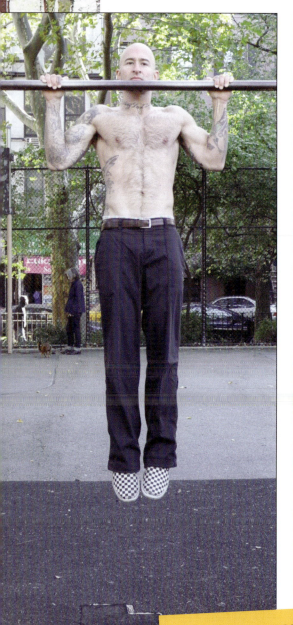
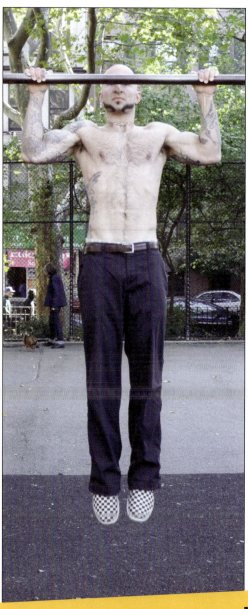
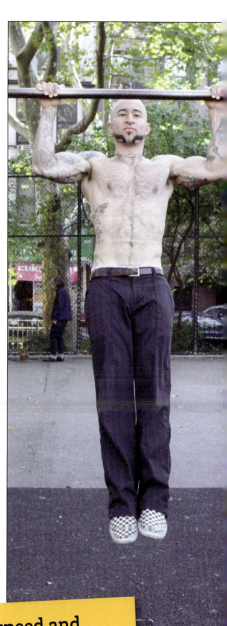

Think of lowering yourself at a normal speed and freezing for half of a second every inch of the way down.

Raising the Bar

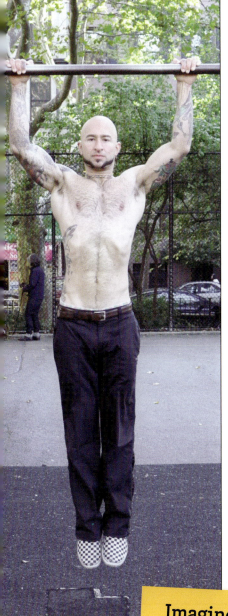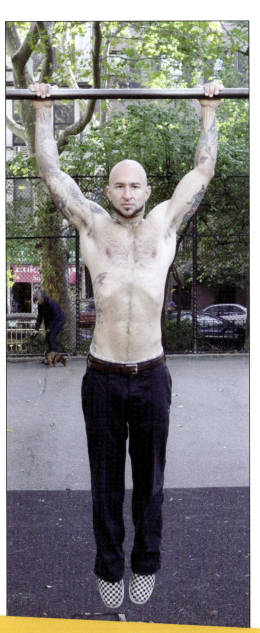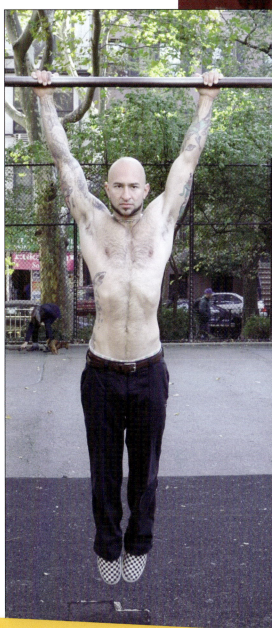

Imagine a photographer is trying to take a series of photos and you need to be still during each shot.

Dead Hangs

If you are not strong enough to do a flex hang or a negative yet, your first objective is simply to get a feel for hanging from the bar. This will build grip strength and work your lats and shoulders isometrically. With some practice, you should be able to work to a flex hang fairly quickly. Even once you can perform flex hangs and controlled negatives, it is still helpful to practice dead hangs at the end of your training session when your arms have gotten too fatigued to do more negatives.

When you perform a dead hang, avoid shrugging your shoulders. Think about keeping your chest up while pulling your shoulder blades down and back. This is both safer and more effective.

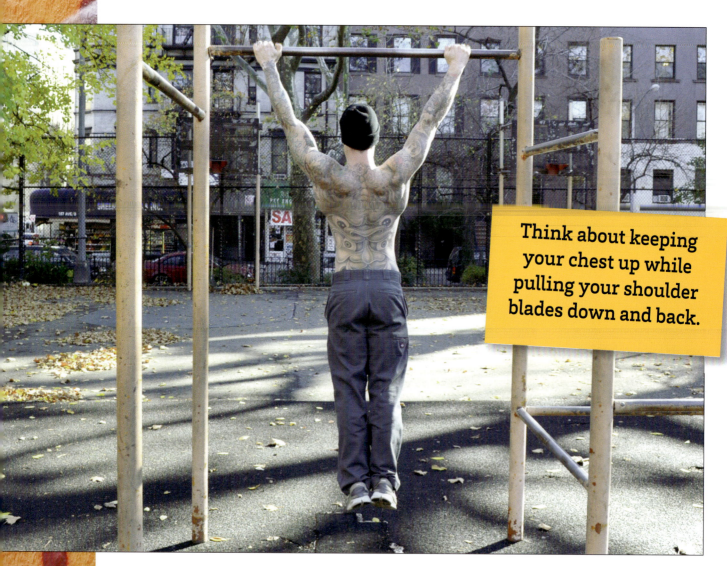

Think about keeping your chest up while pulling your shoulder blades down and back.

It is important to note that overweight and obese individuals will have a much harder time with all bodyweight exercises, especially bar calisthenics. Once you get your body fat percentage into a healthy range, pull-ups (and life in general!) will become much more manageable.

Australian Pull-ups: Down Under the Bar

The Australian pull-up (or bodyweight row as it's sometimes known) is a great exercise for someone who is working their way up to a standard pull-up. The Australian involves getting "down under" a bar that is a little above waist height, with your feet resting on the ground. Keep a straight line from your heels to the back of your head as you squeeze your shoulder blades together and pull your chest to the bar. Novices may choose to bend their knees and push gently with their heels in order to give their arms assistance if needed. When you get a little more comfortable with this exercise you can angle your heels to the floor with your feet pointed up and your legs straight. Like a standard pull-up, the Australian tends to be a bit easier with an underhand grip, though I believe there is more benefit for beginners to practice the overhand version once they are strong enough.

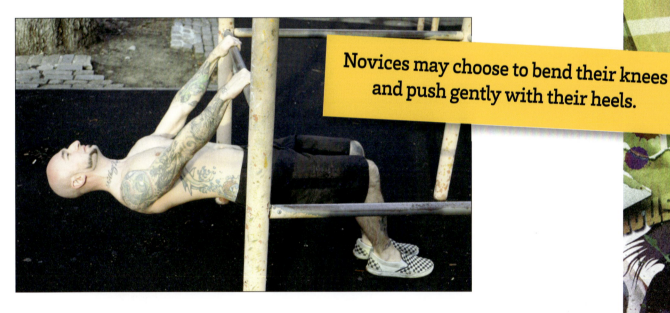

> **Novices may choose to bend their knees and push gently with their heels.**

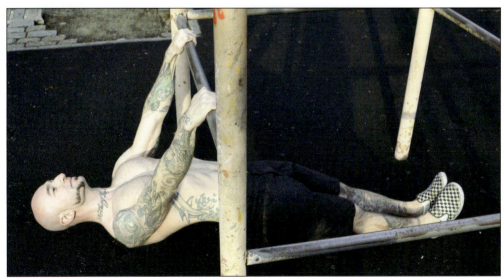

Just like the dead hang, be sure that you are not shrugging your shoulders up when performing Australians. You want to pull your shoulder blades down and back - never up. This is the case for all pull-ups. Start getting in the habit of doing this right away - it's the most common error I see people make when performing these moves.

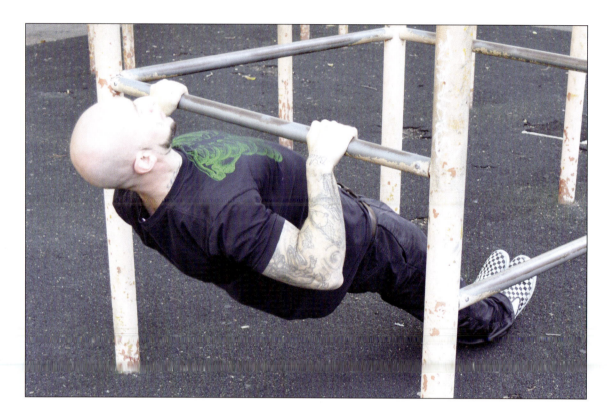

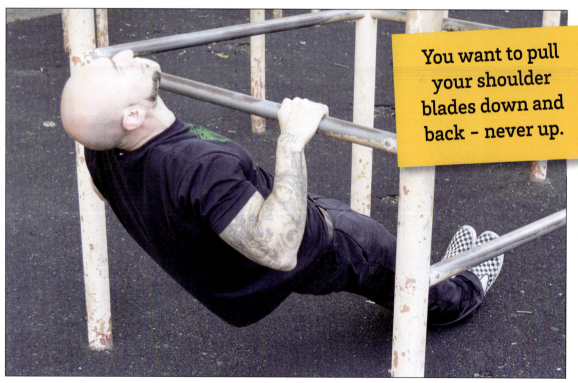

> You want to pull your shoulder blades down and back – never up.

Chin-ups

Once you are strong enough to do lot of Australian pull-ups and negative pull-ups, you will be ready to start working on chin-ups. As with the flex hang, it is easier for beginners to start with an underhand grip first.

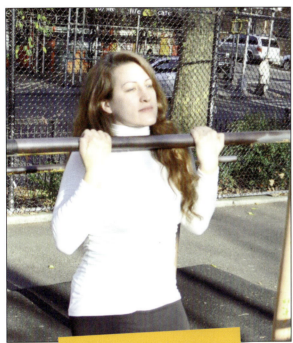

Chin it to win it.

If you've gotten pretty good with Aussies but you still can't manage a single pull-up, here's something to practice. Get under the bar with your feet resting on a step or bench (or use a lower bar if you have access) so you can grab the bar overhead with your feet flat and elbows slightly bent. From here, you can assist yourself by jumping into the pull-up. Jump as hard as you can and in time you will be able to initiate the movement with a smaller jump and eventually without jumping at all.

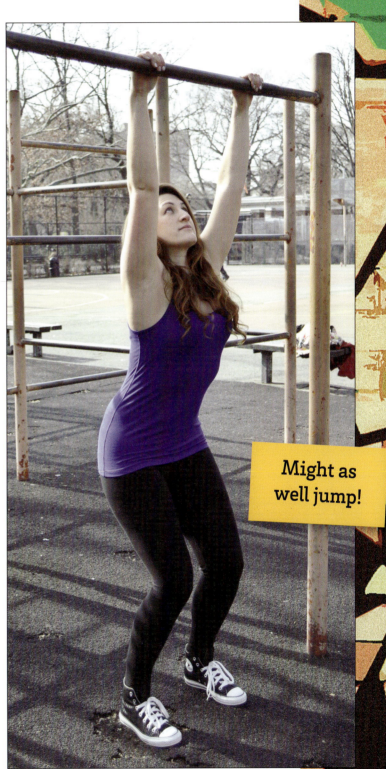

Might as well jump!

Getting an Assist:

Having a trainer or training partner to spot you can be very helpful while you are learning to do pull-ups, just make sure they don't do too much of the work for you. I find it best to spot someone on their back rather than holding their feet as it allows me to adjust how much help I am giving them.

You might need a little extra help initiating the movement as well as during the last few inches, but the idea is for the spotter to make you really work for it. It is important to discuss this with your workout partner to make sure you are on the same page. If they're giving you too much help, you'll never build up the strength to do it on your own.

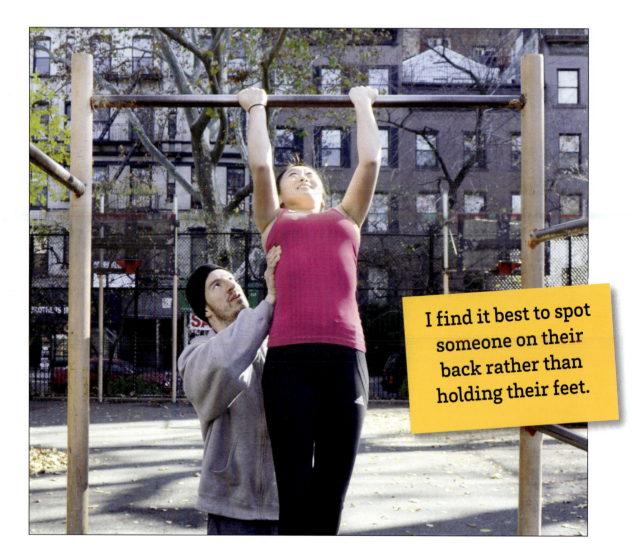

I find it best to spot someone on their back rather than holding their feet.

Raising the Bar

One more thing, steer clear of assisted pull-up machines that allow you to rest your body on a platform. They provide too much stability and therefore do not require the core strength needed for an actual pull-up. You'll never build to the real deal with this type of machine. Beginners who don't have a spotter are better off practicing pull-ups using a rubber exercise band.

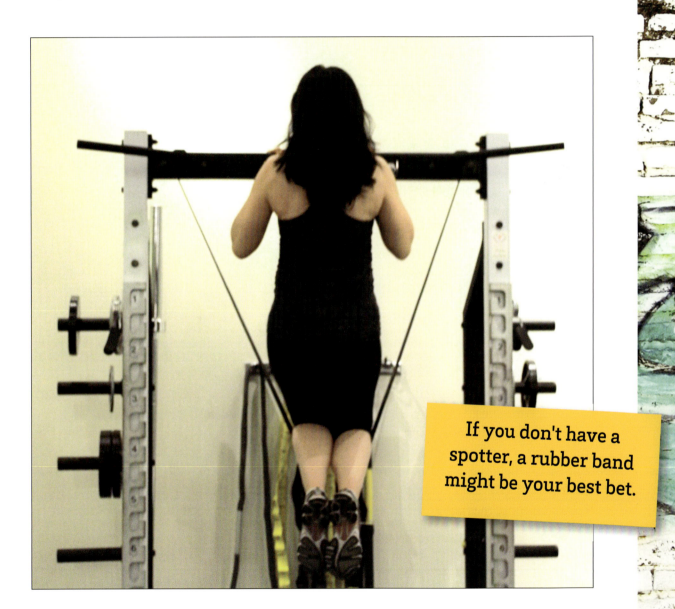

If you don't have a spotter, a rubber band might be your best bet.

All Pull, No Bull

After you can do a dead hang chin-up, you may begin training for the classic pull-up (overhand grip just wider than shoulder width). You may need to go back a step and practice flex hangs and negatives with an overhand grip in order to prepare your body for a pull-up, as you won't be able to use your biceps as much as you do with the chin-up.

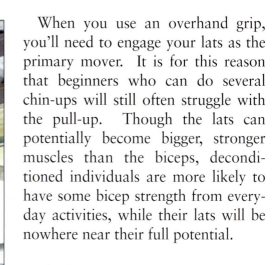

When you use an overhand grip, you'll need to engage your lats as the primary mover. It is for this reason that beginners who can do several chin-ups will still often struggle with the pull-up. Though the lats can potentially become bigger, stronger muscles than the biceps, deconditioned individuals are more likely to have some bicep strength from every-day activities, while their lats will be nowhere near their full potential.

The key to overcoming this is not to think of the pull up simply as an arm exercise. Your lats are doing the bulk of the work, followed by your shoulders, chest and abs. Rather than simply focusing on pulling your chin past the bar, think about squeezing your whole body tight and pulling your elbows into your sides while keeping your chest up. This will help you recruit more of your muscles. Remember the concept of total body tension discussed earlier. When you are performing a pull-up you must keep your body rigid. The pull-up is actually one of the best abdominal exercises out there. Beginners are often surprised at how sore a day of pull-up training can leave their abs. I give the credit for my defined midsection to pull-ups and hanging leg raises (more on those in chapter 3). I haven't done crunches in years and I have no plans of ever doing them again.

RAISING THE BAR

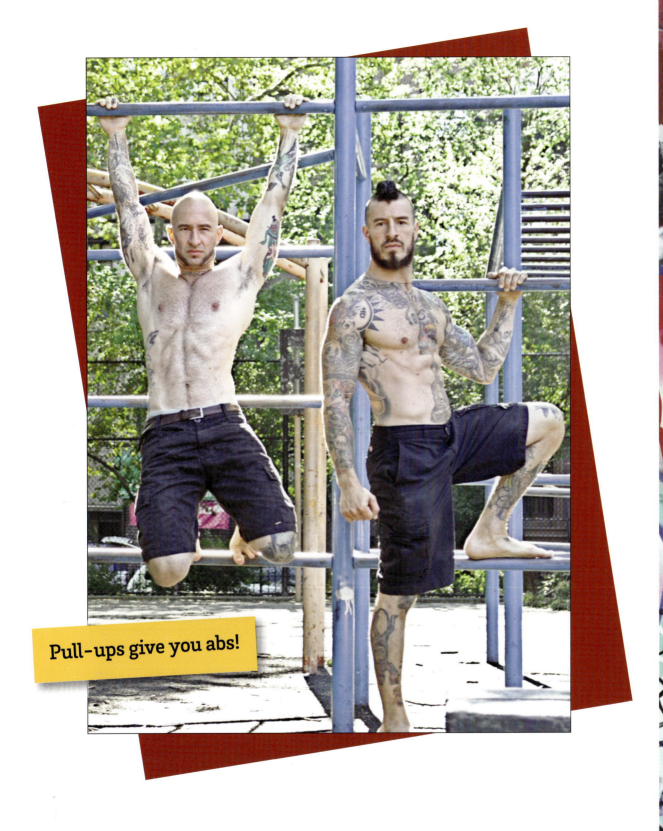

Pull-ups give you abs!

Bars and Grips

The best bar to train on is a plain-old no-frills straight metal bar. You don't need rubberized handles and you don't need ergonomic angled grips. The less fancy your pull-up bar is, the better. My favorite bars to train on are the one at Tompkins Square Park in NYC and the one that my brother Danny and I built in his backyard in Brooklyn.

When training pull-ups, bear in mind that the thickness of the bar will effect your strength. Pull-ups on thick bars require increased grip output and will fatigue your muscles quicker, so I would suggest beginners start with thinner bars. However, for an intermediate or high level trainee, thick bars can be beneficial for building grip strength.

Most standard pull-up bars are one inch thick. The bars at Tompkins Square Park are one and a half inches thick. The bars my brother Danny and I built in his backyard are two inches thick. We train hard in Brooklyn!

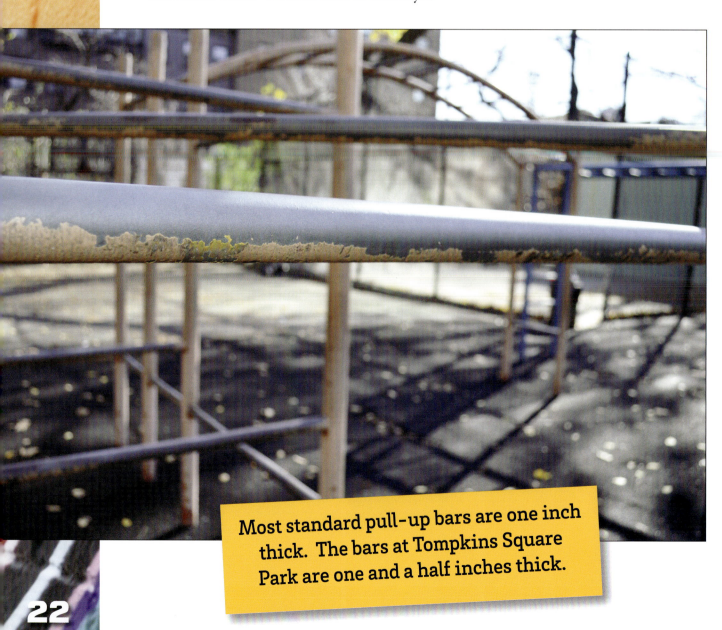

Most standard pull-up bars are one inch thick. The bars at Tompkins Square Park are one and a half inches thick.

Raising the Bar

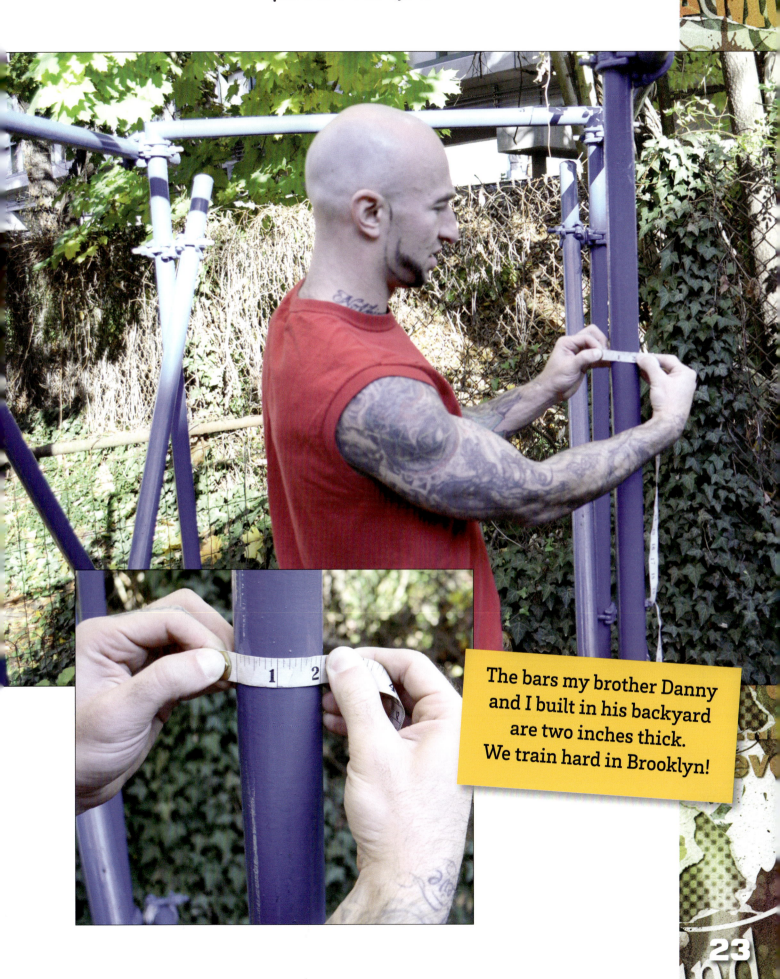

The bars my brother Danny and I built in his backyard are two inches thick. We train hard in Brooklyn!

Hook it Up

When you grip a fat bar in the normal wrap-around fashion, your thumb won't make it all the way around unless you have very large hands. For this reason, the hook grip will allow most people to get a more solid grasp. Hooking your thumb against your index finger lets you keep your hand together tightly. Your grip is stronger this way. I actually suggest practicing with a hook grip regardless of the thickness of your bar. A quick look at these photos should show you what I mean:

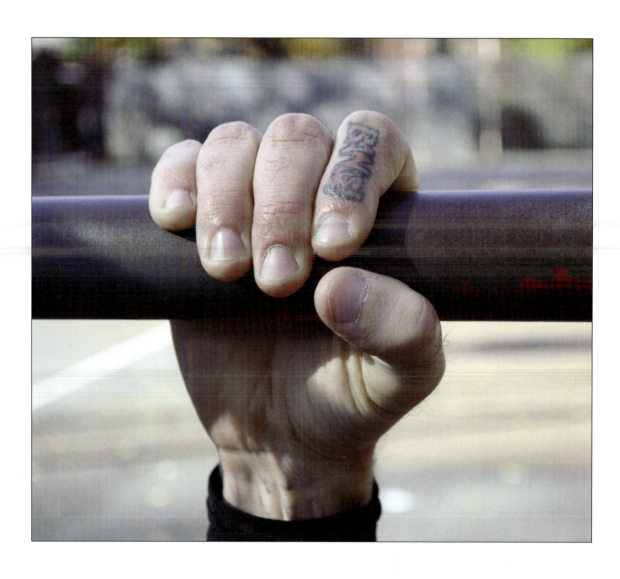

Though supinated (underhand) and pronated (overhand) grips are the two most common ones used for pull-ups, there are other types of grips that you can experiment with. Using two bars that are parallel to each other instead of one straight bar allows you to put your hands into a neutral position with your palms facing each other. Some people will find this to be a nice intermediary step between the underhand and overhand grips. We all have our unique strengths and weakness, so I urge you to practice each of these three primary grips (underhand, overhand and neutral). With repetition, the pulling power of the lats will eventually surpass that of the biceps, which will help even out the disparity of difficulty between various grips.

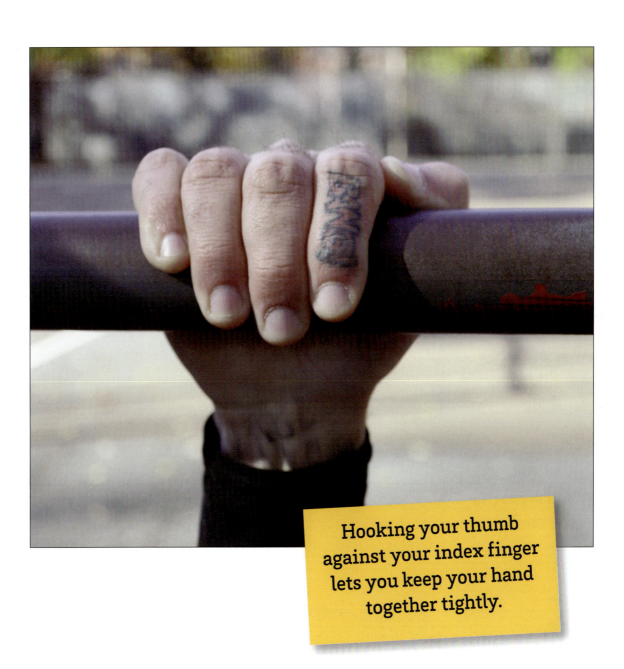

Hooking your thumb against your index finger lets you keep your hand together tightly.

Strength in Numbers

Try to avoid the temptation to move onto harder exercises until you can perform at least ten reps of the previous movement. Even once you can do twenty or more reps of a given exercise in one set, it is still worthwhile to keep training that exercise. I'll always keep pull-ups and dips in my workouts.

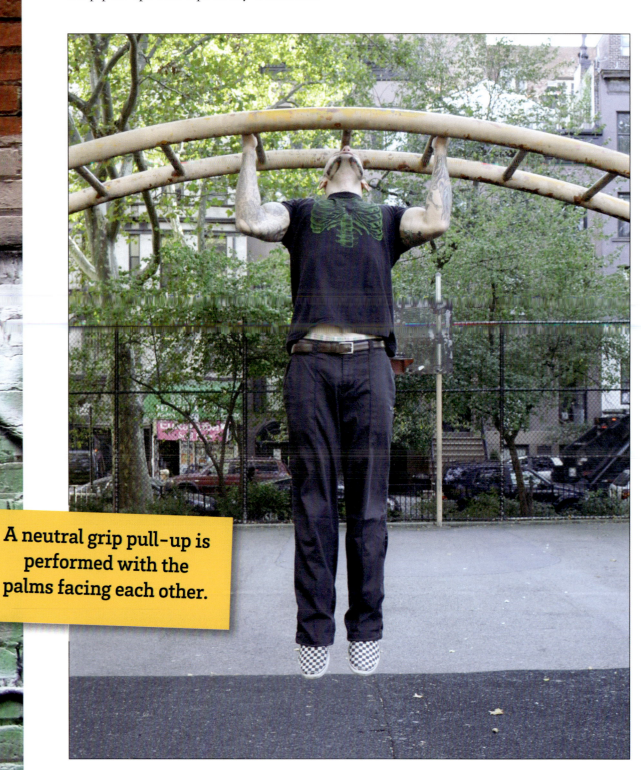

A neutral grip pull-up is performed with the palms facing each other.

Raising the Bar

The idea that strength and endurance are on opposite sides of the spectrum is not always the case. The guys who perform feats like one arm pull-ups and front lever holds are often the same guys who can do 25+ pull-ups in one set. Never stop training the basics - pull-ups should be a part of everyone's training regimen. Without a solid foundation, even the tallest building would easily crumble.

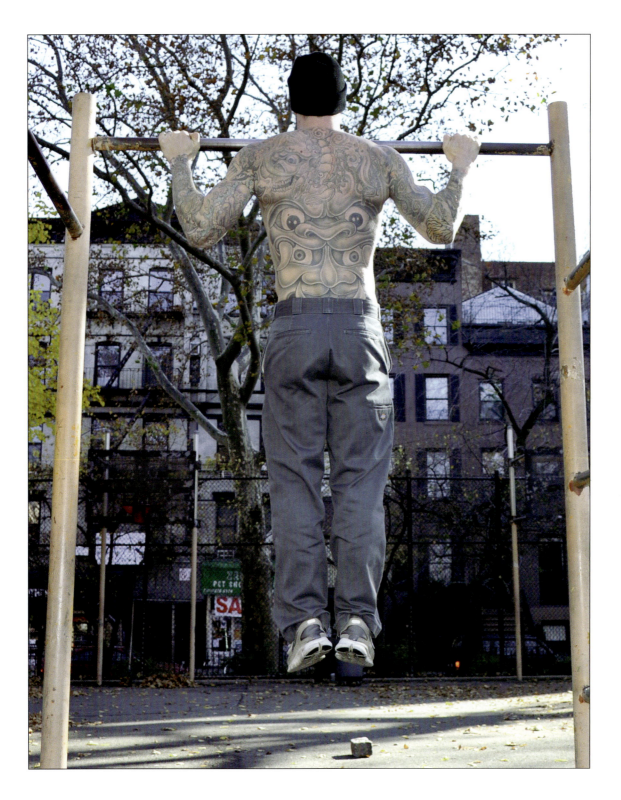

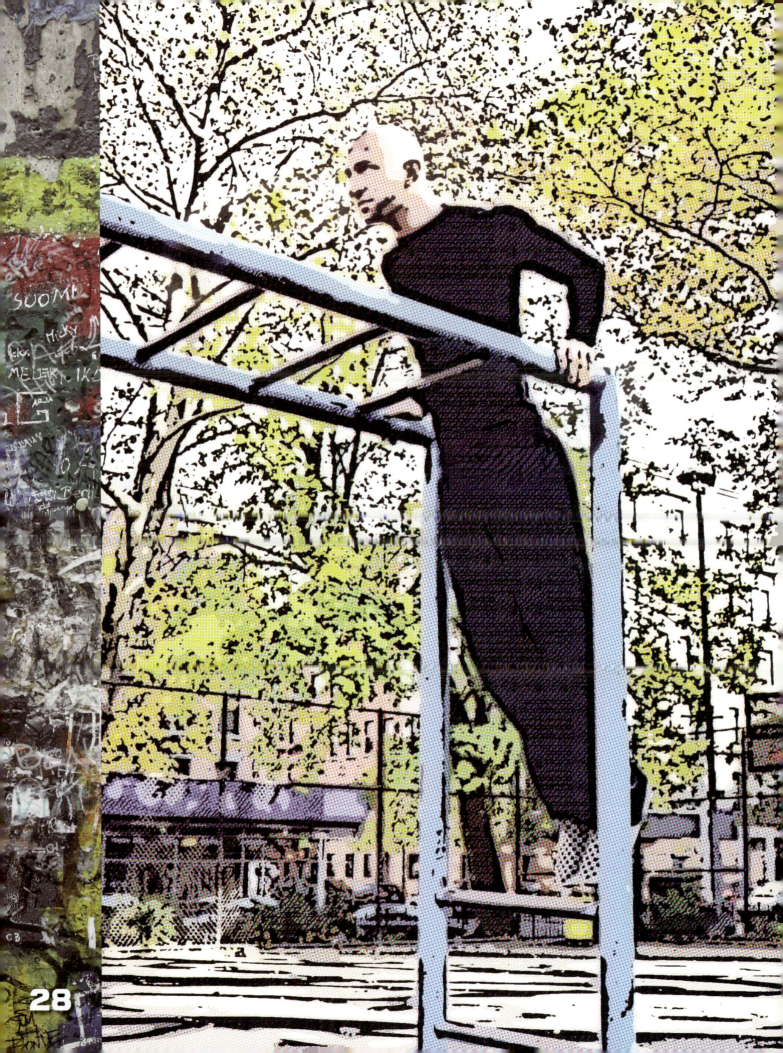

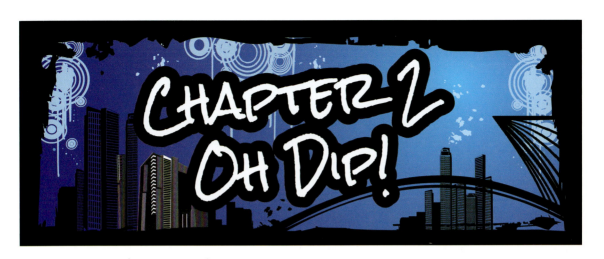

Chapter 2
Oh Dip!

"Simplicity is the ultimate sophistication."
−Leonardo Da Vinci

Though bar training is a simple, stripped-down way of exercising, there's still a lot going on. So far, we've pretty much only talked about the straight bar. However, the parallel bars are another key component of bar calisthenics. One of my most vivid adolescent memories is the first time I ever attempted a triceps dip on parallel bars. It was my freshman year of high school and I had just started to explore the wonderful world of working out. I signed up to take weight training my second semester that year and there was a dip station in the weight room, so I decided to give it a go. In theory, the parallel bar dip is a very simple exercise, so I felt confident approaching the bars. I grabbed the handles, jumped into the top position and braced myself for my first dip.

Once I began lowering down however, everything suddenly changed. I felt like someone had punched me hard in the sternum and rather than being able to press myself back up, I instead fell to the ground and recoiled in pain.   At that point I was pretty sure I would NEVER be able to do a single dip on the bars. The few kids in gym class who could do one suddenly seemed like super-human deities.

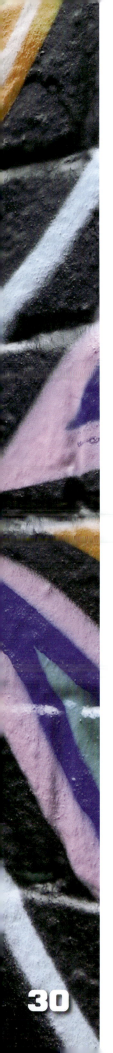

Raising the Bar

I didn't let that early experience stop me from trying again, however, and a few weeks later, I got my first real dip – it was a very exciting time! I've done a lot of dips since then and learned a lot of different variations. Dips are a great exercise and there are endless ways to keep them fresh and challenging. Pretty much any time you use your arms to press your body while in an upright position, it's a dip.

Keep in mind that while dips emphasize the triceps, they also work your chest, shoulders and core muscles.

Low Bar Dips

A great way for novices to work up towards full dips (and avoid the humiliation I felt after my first try) is by first practicing with the feet resting on the ground. This is most commonly done by placing your hands on a bench or a low bar held behind the back, with your hands in a pronated grip.

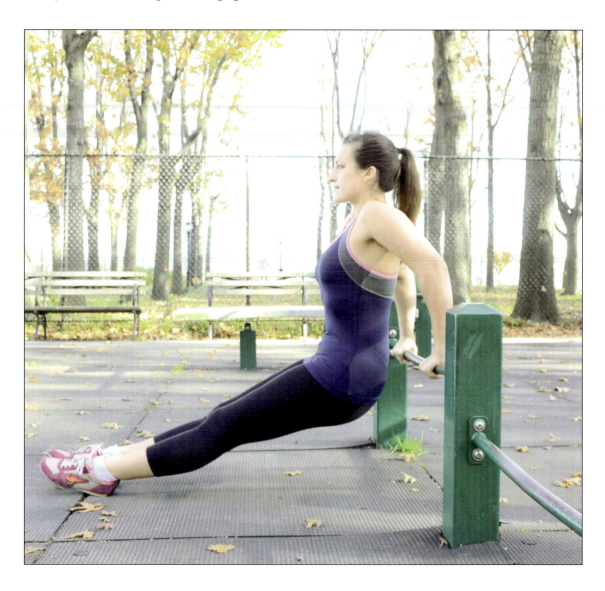

Raising the Bar

Beginners should start with their knees bent and feet flat on the floor. This allows you to push gently with your legs in order to give your arms some assistance. Make sure to hold your chest high. Don't allow your shoulders to shrug upwards.

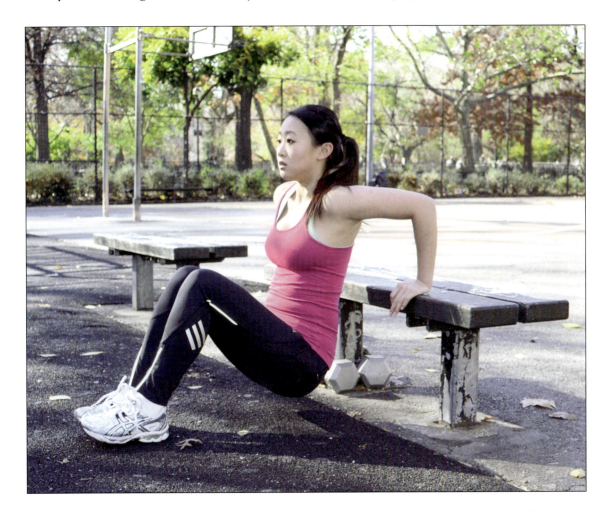

When low bar dips with your feet flat become easy, you can progress to doing them with your legs straight and your toes pointed up. Let your legs relax and allow your hips to hang down right below your shoulders. Your arms will have to do more of the work this way.

It might take a lot of practice for some people to get the feel for how to perform this move correctly. It is common for beginners to shrug their shoulders, lean over and hardly bend their elbows at all. Most of the time, these people have no idea that they are doing it until someone points it out and guides them through the proper range of motion. I can't tell you how many times I've literally had to hold someone's arms and physically bend their elbow for them to perform the correct movement pattern. It's always helpful to videotape yourself in order to objectively assess your form. Nowadays everyone has a camcorder in their phone, so it shouldn't be too hard.

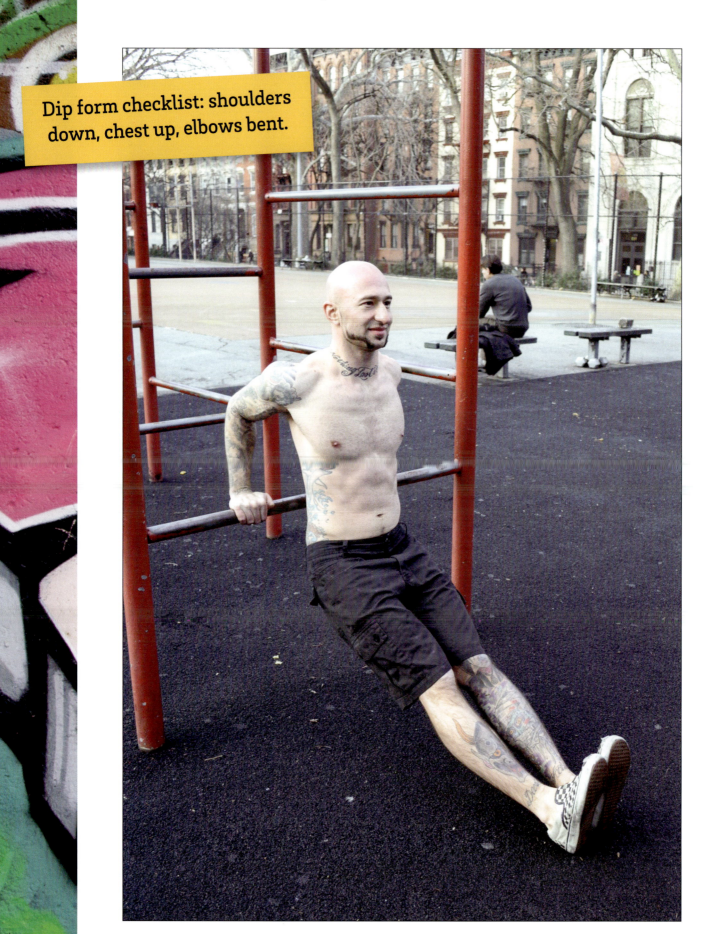

Dip form checklist: shoulders down, chest up, elbows bent.

RAISING THE BAR

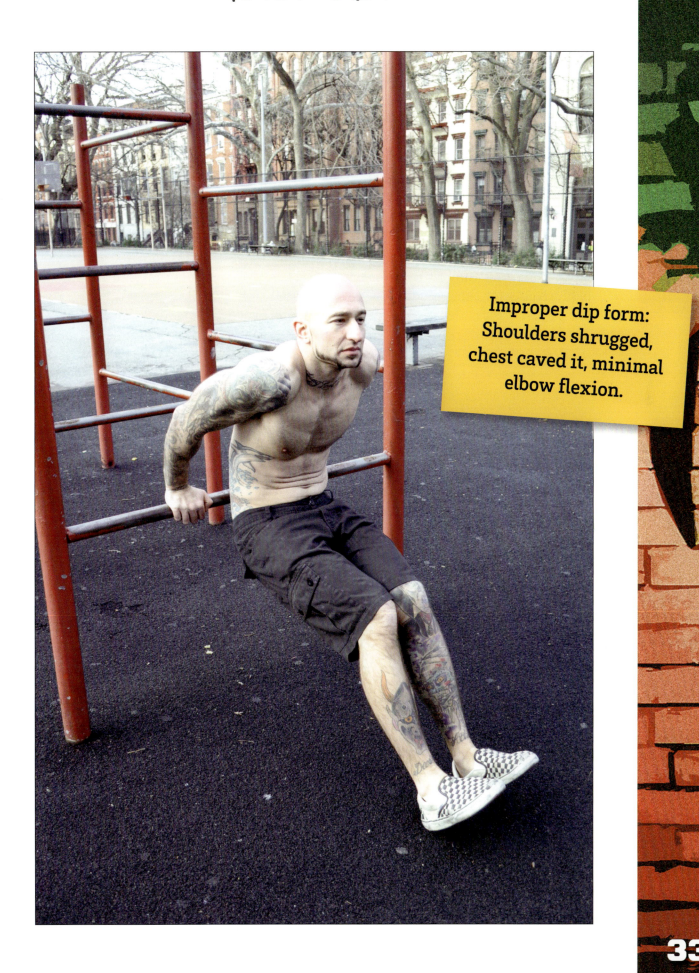

Improper dip form: Shoulders shrugged, chest caved it, minimal elbow flexion.

Raising the Bar

The jump from low bar dips to full parallel bar dips can be a big hurdle. You'll likely need to be able to do at least 20 on the low bar before you'll manage even one dip on the parallel bars. Some may get there quickly (young men especially), but it will take longer for others. Don't be in a rush to get to the finish. One step at a time, one rep at a time.

Parallel Bar Dips

Once you can comfortably perform many dips with your feet resting on the ground you will be ready to attempt the real deal. The parallel bar set-up is the gold standard for the triceps dip exercise. Like pull-ups (and most of the exercises in this book for that matter), dips will be more difficult for women than they are for men. They are still amongst the best exercises for either gender.

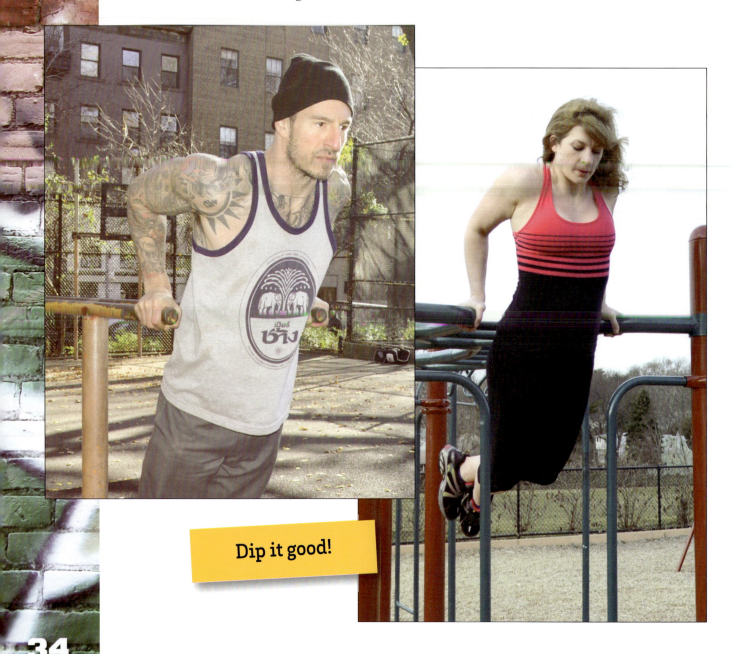

Dip it good!

Raising the Bar

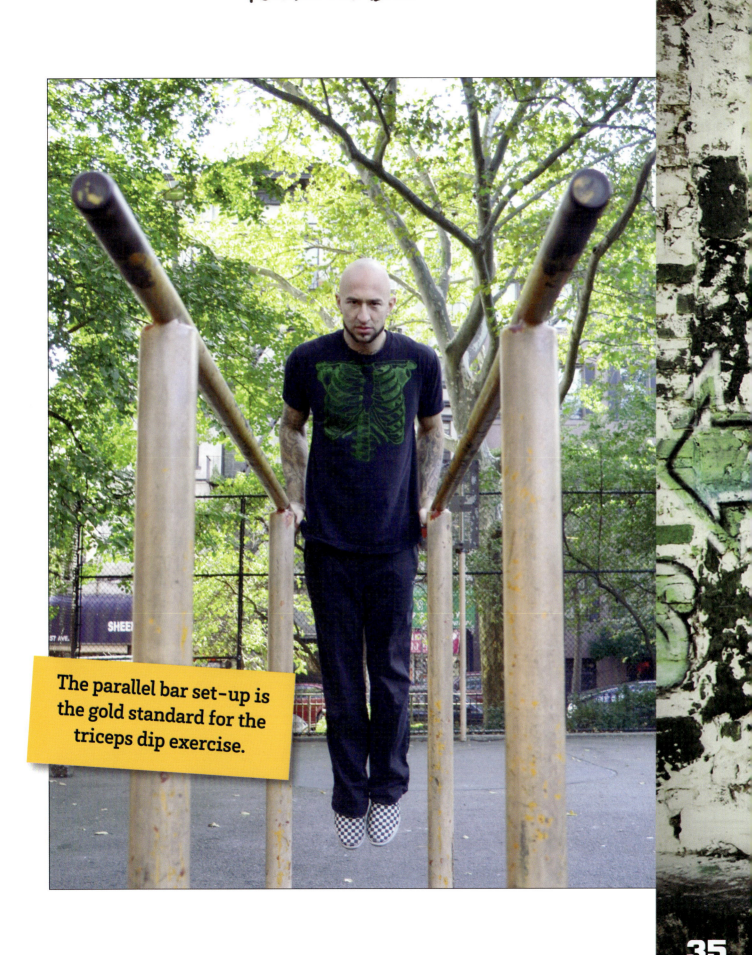

The parallel bar set-up is the gold standard for the triceps dip exercise.

RAISING THE BAR

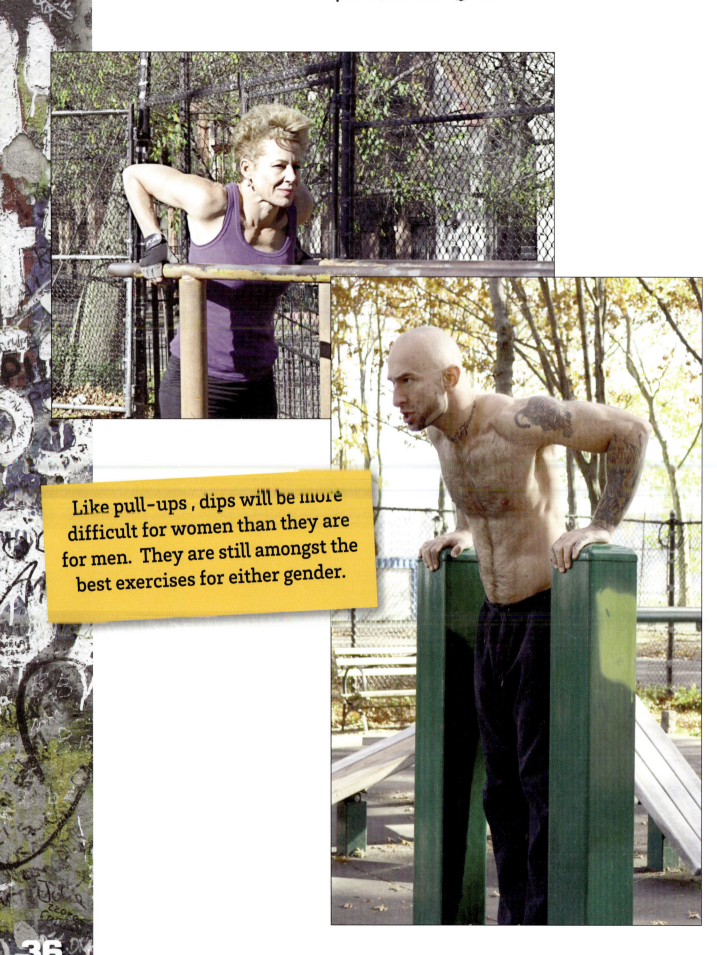

Like pull-ups, dips will be more difficult for women than they are for men. They are still amongst the best exercises for either gender.

Raising the Bar

When performing parallel bar dips, you'll need to tilt forward at the torso. Your elbows should stay more or less over your hands, so your shoulders will wind up in front of them. You can vary the degree to which you do this, and doing so can change the emphasis. The more you lean forward the more you are working your chest. The more upright you stay, the more you work your triceps and core. Trying to stay totally vertical is not advised, however, as doing so can put unnecessary strain on your shoulders. Unless you're really, really strong.

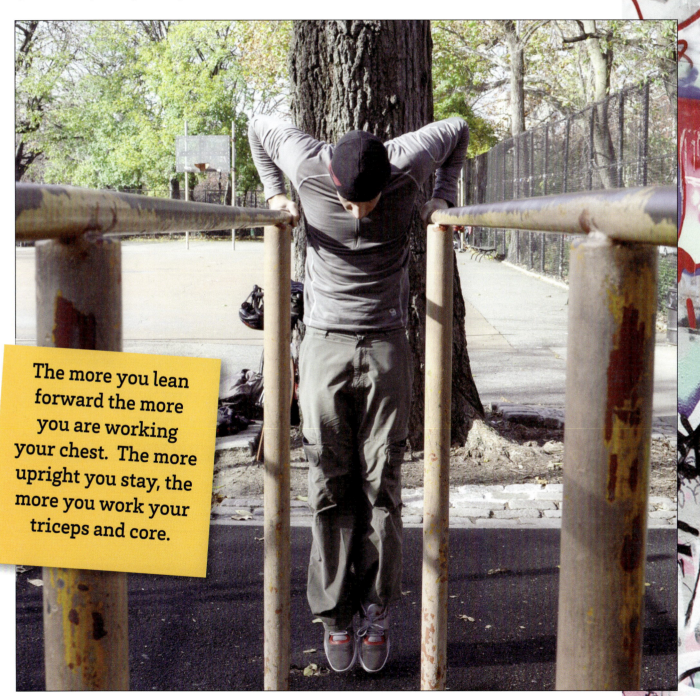

The more you lean forward the more you are working your chest. The more upright you stay, the more you work your triceps and core.

Raising the Bar

It is worth noting that the distance between the bars and thickness of the grip will effect the difficulty of the exercise. Beginners are better off using thinner bars spaced fairly far apart (20-24 inches), while closer bars (anything closer than 18 or 19 inches is pretty narrow) will provide increased difficulty.

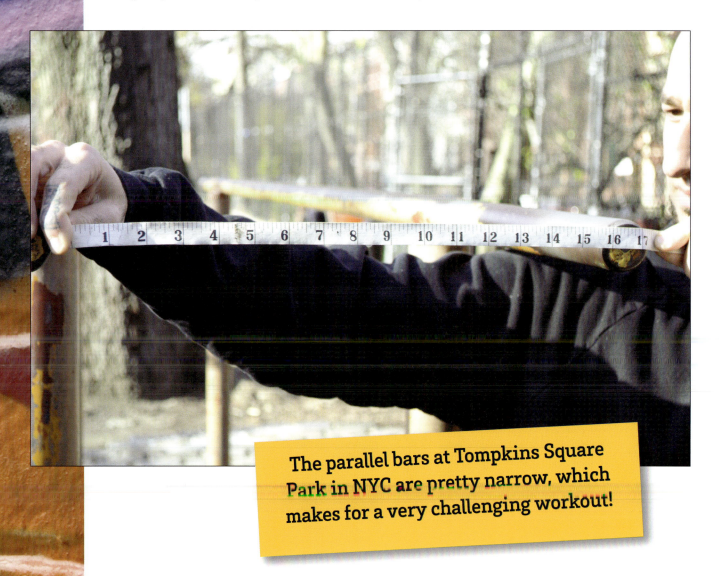

The parallel bars at Tompkins Square Park in NYC are pretty narrow, which makes for a very challenging workout!

Straight Bar Dips

Straight bar dips are another challenging and worthwhile variation. As the name implies, the straight bar dip is performed with both hands on a single straight bar positioned in front of the body. When you do a parallel bar dip, you dip in between the bars, but when you dip on a straight bar, your body must move around the bar. As you lower yourself down, you'll need to reach your legs out in front a bit to keep balance.

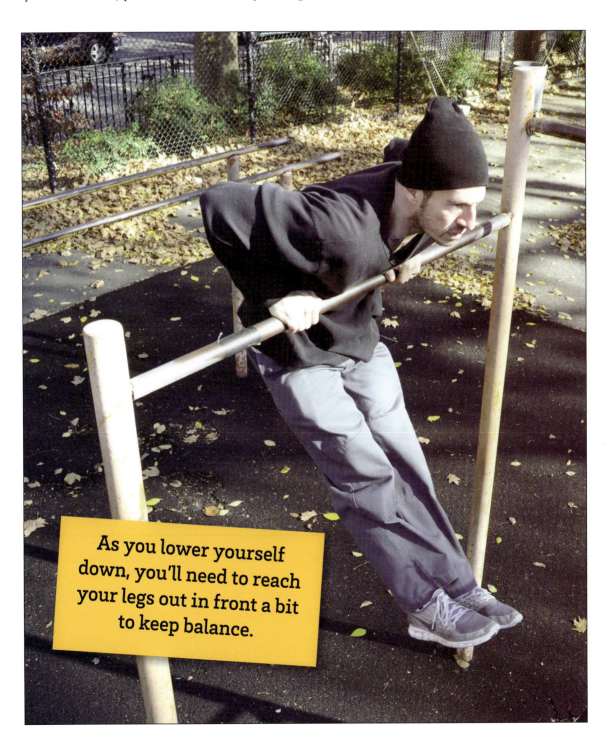

As you lower yourself down, you'll need to reach your legs out in front a bit to keep balance.

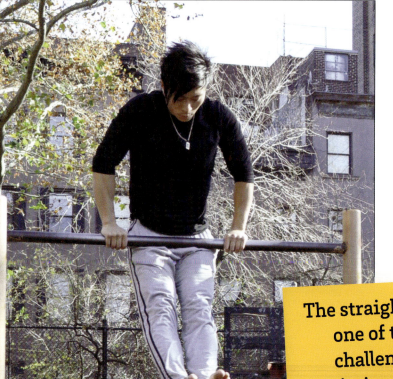

The straight bar dip is one of the more challenging dip variations and one of the most specific precursors to the muscle-up. You should start working on these once you can do a few reps on the parallel bars.

> The straight bar dip is one of the more challenging dip variations and one of the most specific precursors to the muscle-up.

Perpendicular Bar Dips

You can also split the difference between the parallel bars and the straight bar by practicing your dips on two perpendicular bars. Feel free to get creative with everyday scenarios if you don't have access to formal workout equipment.

Dips on the perpendicular bars and parallel bars are very similar, though they each have their own nuances. Just like with parallel bars, playing around with how far forward you lean can effect the subtleties of muscle recruitment. Lean forward for more chest, stay upright for more triceps and abs. The perpendicular bar set-up can allow you to stay more upright without the potential shoulder strain. Just make sure you are strong enough to handle this variation before you start trying to rep out.

RAISING THE BAR

You can do perpendicular bar dips in lots of creative places!

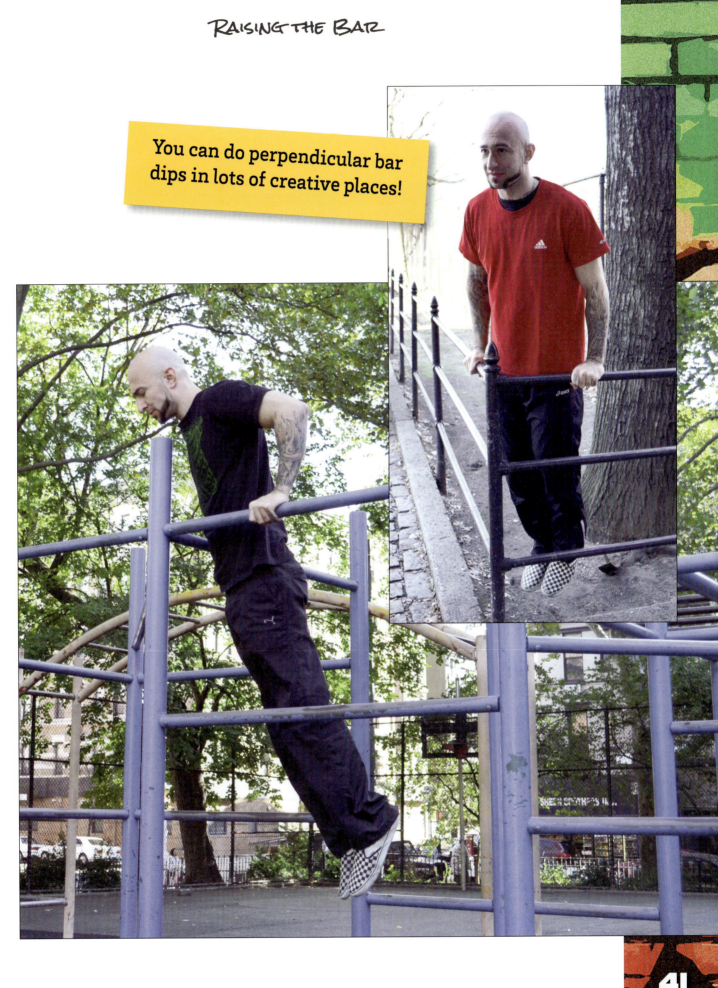

41

Korean Dips

A Korean dip is a behind the back dip on a high bar. It's almost like the low bar dip I talked about earlier, except your feet are in the air!

This is one of the hardest dip variations, so I suggest getting very comfortable with the others before attempting the Korean dip. You should be able to perform at least fifteen consecutive parallel or perpendicular bar dips first. Because it is difficult to control your body from this angle, you'll really need to focus on engaging your abs and lower back muscles to stabilize. It also helps to keep your hamstrings and glutes contracted. Having the bar behind you can give your shoulders a deep stretch as well, so make sure you are warmed up. The Korean dip is really a full body exercise.

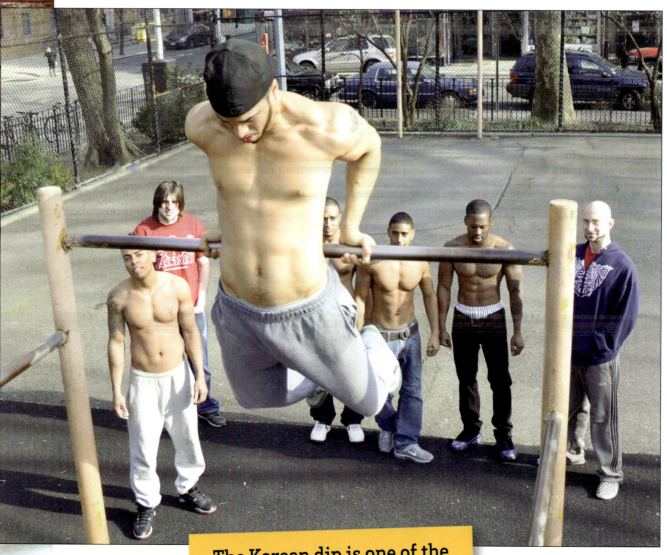

The Korean dip is one of the hardest dip variations.

Hinge Dips

Also known as a Russian dip, the hinge dip starts out like a standard parallel bar dip. When you reach the bottom of the normal range of motion, shift your weight back onto your elbows, putting your forearms in contact with the bars. Then shift your weight back onto your hands and press yourself up.

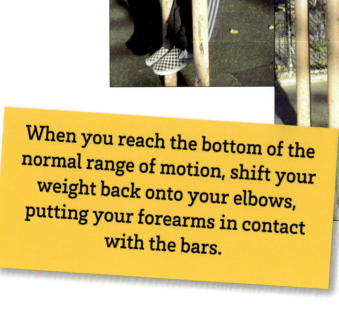

> When you reach the bottom of the normal range of motion, shift your weight back onto your elbows, putting your forearms in contact with the bars.

Sliding Hinge Dips

To make hinge dips even more difficult, you can extend the range of motion by sliding your entire body out until your arms are straight. It's helpful to contract your abs and reach your legs out in front of your trunk when sitting back all the way into a sliding hinge dip. If you let your upper arm come off the bar as you lean back, the exercise will become more difficult. Very advanced practitioners may also be able to perform a forward sliding hinge dip onto the shoulders.

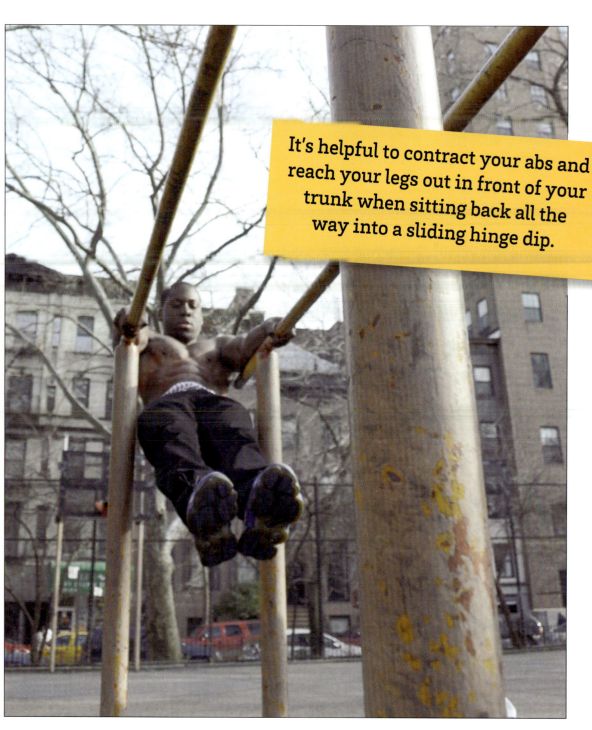

> It's helpful to contract your abs and reach your legs out in front of your trunk when sitting back all the way into a sliding hinge dip.

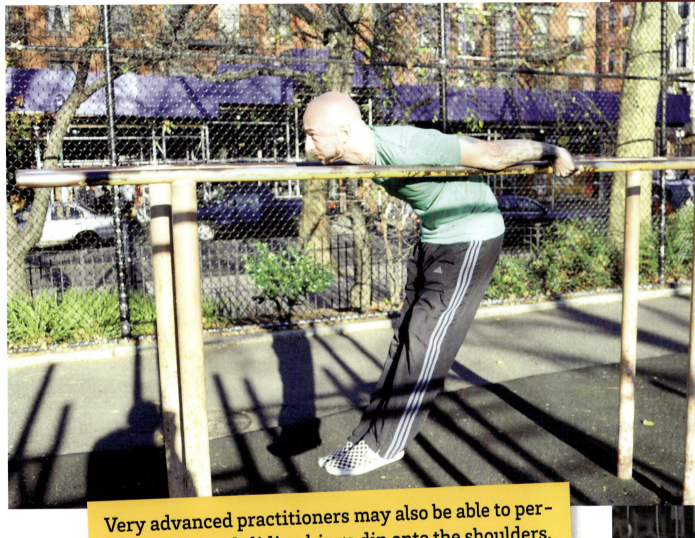

Very advanced practitioners may also be able to perform a forward sliding hinge dip onto the shoulders.

Ply-Oh Dips!

Sometimes referred to as "jump training," the term plyometrics refers to any type of explosive exercise. Any time you get your body airborne you are doing a plyo. Once you're very strong and confident with the previous variations, you can start working on plyometric dips. I'd suggest being able to do at least thirty reps on the parallel bars first.

The idea with a plyo-dip is simply to push your body away from the bar(s) at the top of the rep. Use your hips and put your entire body into it. There's no way to do a slow controlled jump, so move fast and explosively. Eventually you'll get a feel for catching some air and you can experiment with clapping dips and other freestyle variations. The sky is the limit!

Raising the Bar

> Any time you get your body airborne you are doing a plyo.

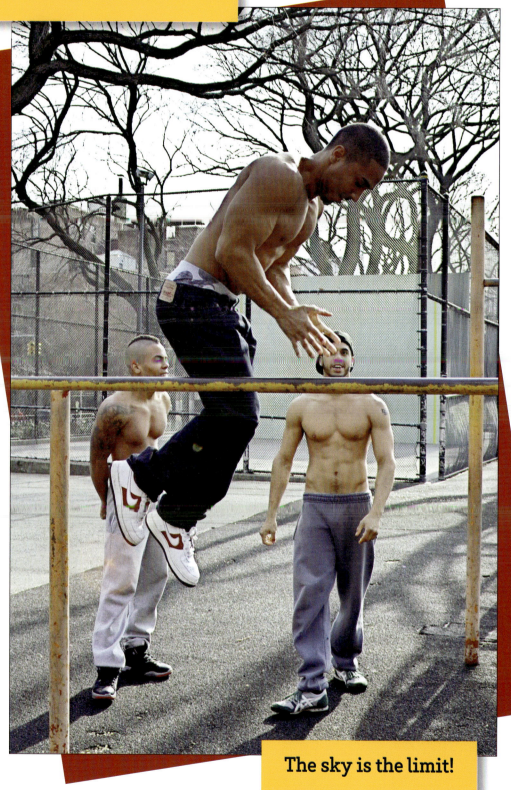

The sky is the limit!

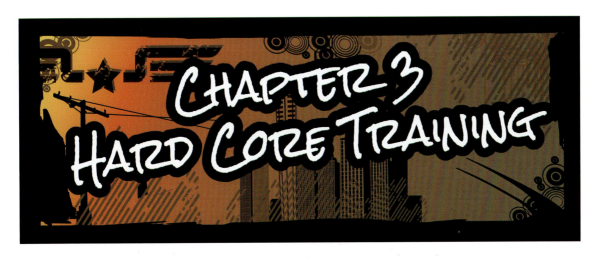

Chapter 3
Hard Core Training

"We are not these bodies.
Let's not get hung up on that."
–George Harrison

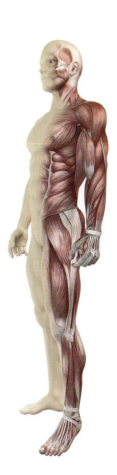

As a functional fitness geek, I had always been curious to observe the inner workings of the human body up close and personal. So when a client of mine gave me tickets to see Bodies: The Exhibition several years ago, I was very excited to finally get that opportunity. Bodies is a display of actual human cadavers stripped of their skin and posed like statues. As anyone who's seen the exhibit knows firsthand, it is quite an unbelievable thing to behold!

As I walked through the museum I observed the preserved bodies of people from all different walks of life. Men and women; athletes and sedentary folk; tall and short; fat and skinny. One thing stood out to me across the board: once these bodies had their flesh removed, each and every one of them had six pack abs underneath. After all, we all have the same anatomical make-up. The same muscles connected by the same tendons and ligaments to the same bones. Though we all look unique and individual, there is a basic formula that remains the same.

The problem for most people is that they have too much fat covering up those beautiful abdominal muscles! No matter how strong your abs

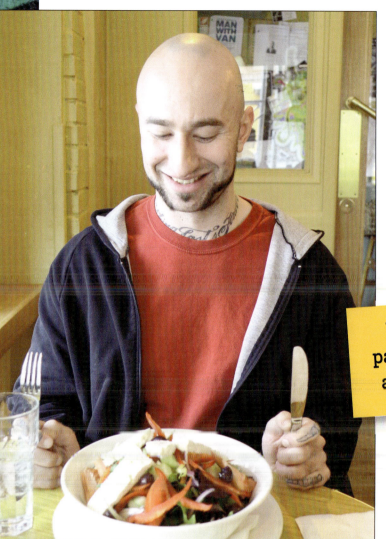

become, you will never see that definition without a low body fat percentage. And while the belly is one of the last places that most people will hold onto fat, the same principle holds true for your whole body. If you're training to get muscle tone, the only way to make that happen is by having a combination of muscle mass and a low body fat percentage. Bar training is a fantastic way to build muscle, but if you want to get a six pack, put that donut down and eat some vegetables.

> If you want to get a six pack, put that donut down and eat some vegetables.

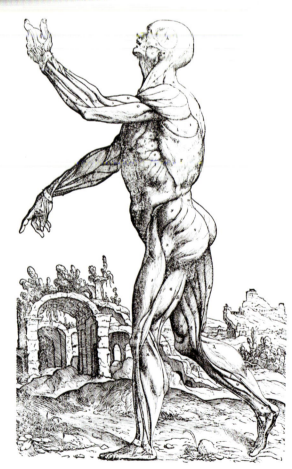

Raising the Bar

The Best Abs Exercises

In order to understand why certain exercises are more effective than others, you must first understand the role that your abs play in the musculoskeletal system. The abs (or rectus abdominis as they are technically known) function primarily as a stabilizer muscle – they keep your torso upright while you're standing, walking or performing other movements. For this reason, the best way to work your abs is to use them to stabilize your trunk in difficult positions. Rather than attempting to isolate them with crunches, I've found it more worthwhile to work my abs in the context of my entire body. You don't need an ab roller or a fancy machine with a weight stack in order to make your abs rock hard either, you just need a bar to hang from. Pull-ups are actually a very effective abdominal exercise on their own. In fact, every single exercise discussed in this book will work your abs! However, additional core exercises will be helpful in your training.

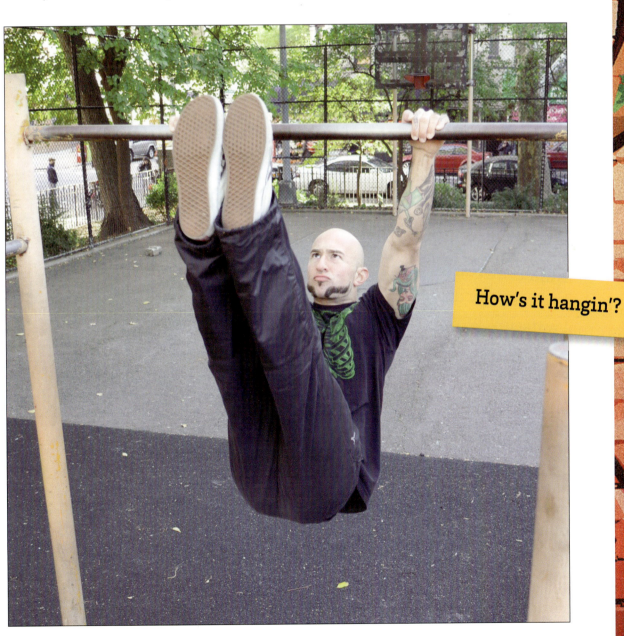

How's it hangin'?

Bent Knee Raise

A full hanging leg raise takes time to work towards. The first step in the progression is the bent knee hanging leg raise. As you begin to raise your knees, think about curling your hips forward to facilitate the movement. Keep in mind that your focus is to engage your abdominal muscles, which are attached to your pelvis, not your legs. Aim to tuck your knees all the way to your chest.

You'll have to go very slowly to stay in control and you'll probably only manage to do a couple of reps your first time out. This is okay; go for quality over quantity and be careful not to swing your body. If you find yourself swinging, try to stop the momentum by touching your feet to the ground in between reps. If you aren't strong enough to do a full hanging knee raise up to your chest, work on doing half hanging knee raises with your knees getting to hip level.

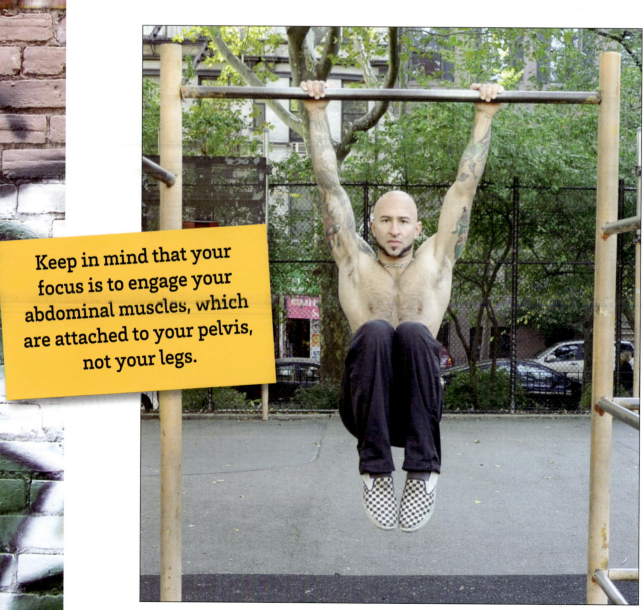

> Keep in mind that your focus is to engage your abdominal muscles, which are attached to your pelvis, not your legs.

Hanging Bicycles

Another variation on the hanging knee raise is the hanging bicycle. Instead of bringing both knees up together, the knees are alternately raised one at a time, like you were riding an imaginary bicycle. This can be a slightly easier variation for anyone struggling to get both legs up together.

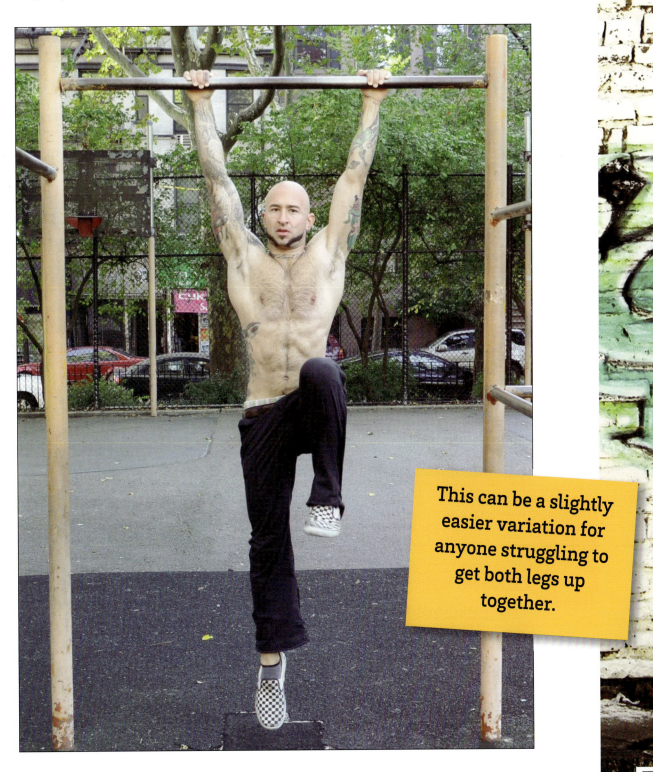

This can be a slightly easier variation for anyone struggling to get both legs up together.

Straight Leg Raise

Once you can do ten consecutive bent-knee leg raises, you're ready to try it with your legs straight. This can be extra challenging for those of us with tight hamstrings. Think about rolling your hips forward as you lift your legs towards the bar. If you have to bend your knees a bit on the way up, this is fine. In time, work towards increasing your flexibility in order to keep your legs straight.

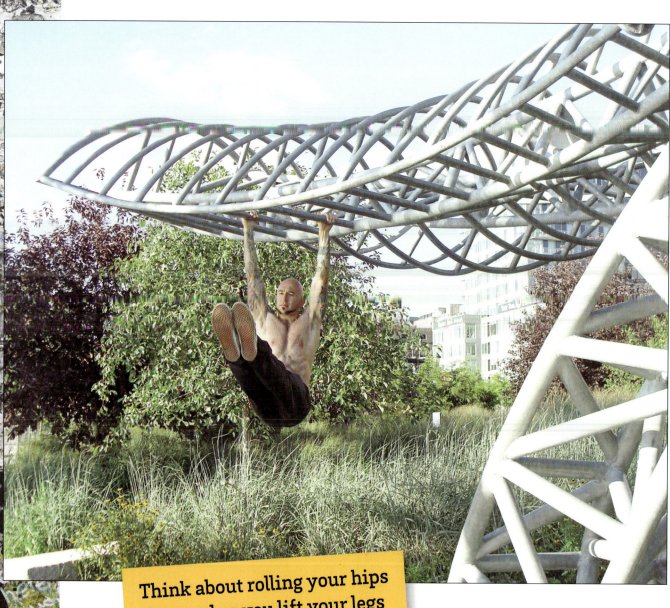

Think about rolling your hips forward as you lift your legs towards the bar.

Circles

After you've gotten comfortable with hanging leg raises, hanging leg circles are the next step in the progression. The idea is to move your legs in a giant circle around your entire body like a clock. Just make sure to do some reps counter-clockwise too! The circle motion will engage your obliques more than a straight leg raise, while still working the rectus abdominis.

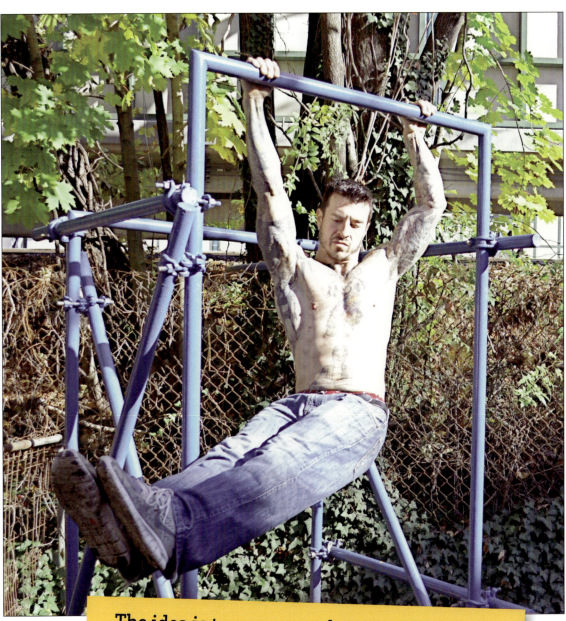

The idea is to move your legs in a giant circle around your entire body like a clock.

Windshield Wipers

Windshield Wipers are another challenging variation on the hanging leg raise. Like the name implies, the windshield wiper involves raising your legs to the bar and twisting from side to side like the windshield wipers of a car. You can think of it as only the top half of the circle. Go slow when performing these movements. Focus on good form rather than how many reps you can do. Three or four full range of motion windshield wipers can be quite difficult if you take your time with them.

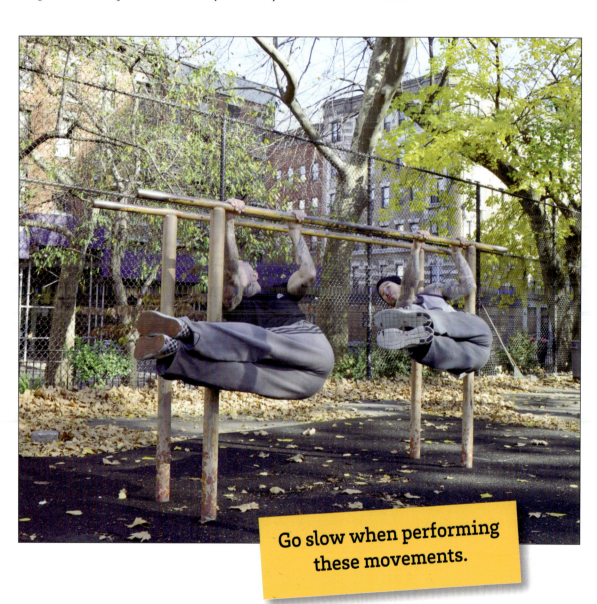

Go slow when performing these movements.

Raising the Bar

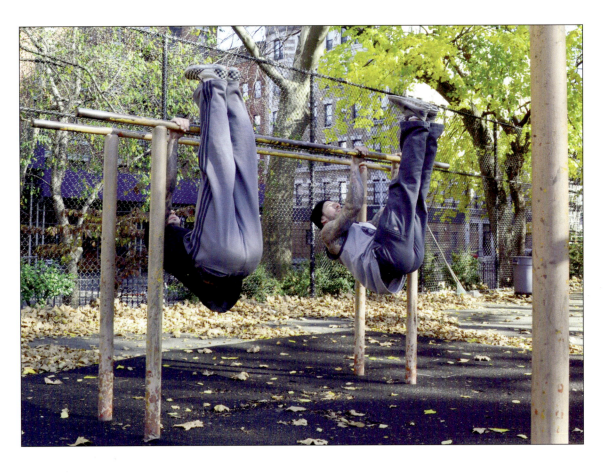

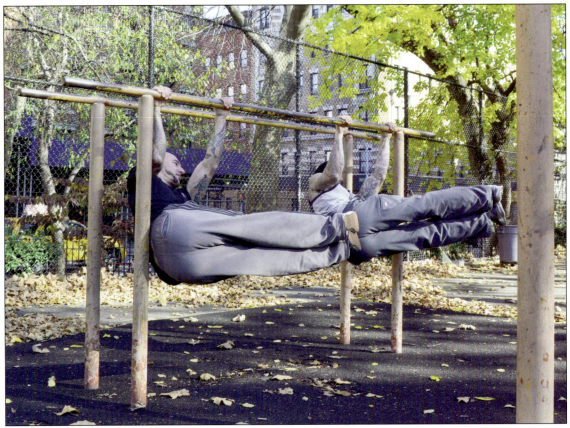

L-Hold

Try doing a hanging leg raise and freezing when your legs are extended at a right angle to your torso. The shape of your body should resemble the letter L. This position is called an L-Hold. (Kind of a no-brainer, right?) Since your legs are extended the furthest from your body during this part of the exercise, it is the most difficult part of the hanging leg raise to hold.

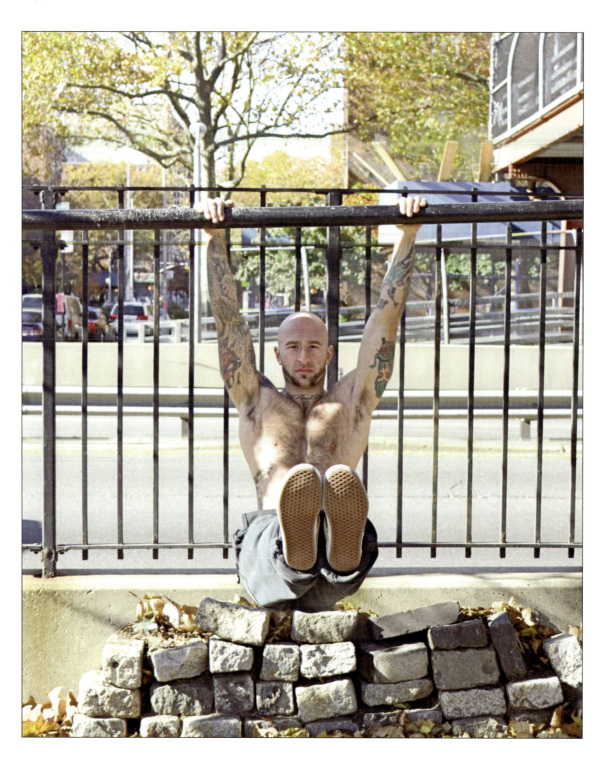

L-Sit:

Though quite effective when executed on the bar, the L-hold is most commonly performed with the hands resting on the ground or holding parallel bars. The same ones that you use for dips are perfect. An L-hold performed in this fashion with the arms alongside the torso and palms below the hips is called an L-sit. How long a person can hold this position is an excellent measure of core strength. Though most commonly seen in gymnastics, the L-sit is a great exercise for anyone who is serious about building core strength. A thirty second L-sit in an excellent indication of a strong core. A minute puts you in an elite category of bodyweight strength.

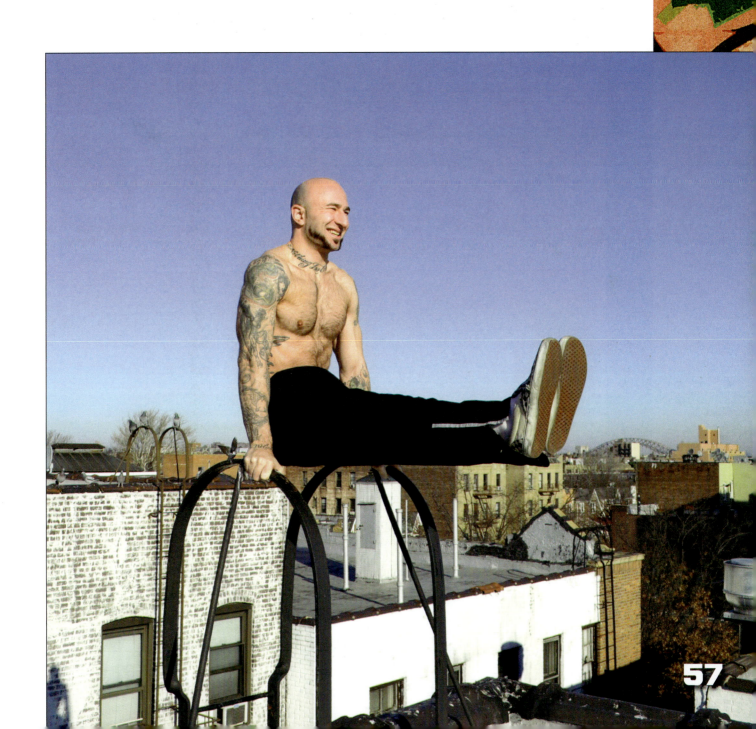

Raising the Bar

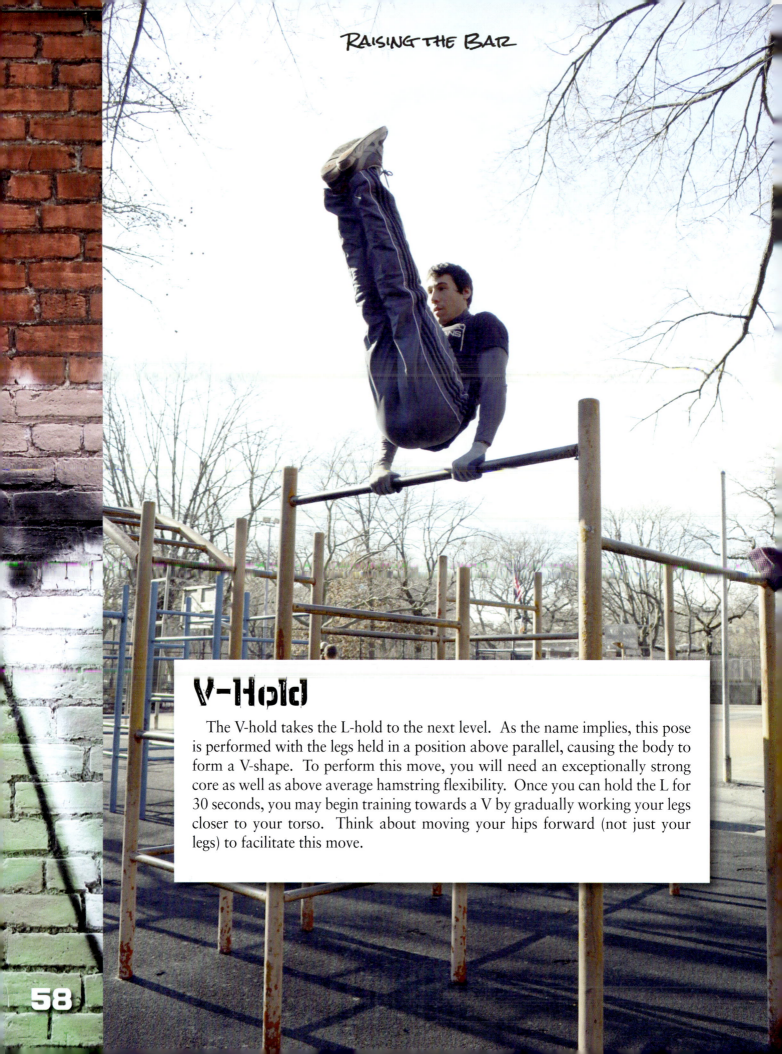

V-Hold

The V-hold takes the L-hold to the next level. As the name implies, this pose is performed with the legs held in a position above parallel, causing the body to form a V-shape. To perform this move, you will need an exceptionally strong core as well as above average hamstring flexibility. Once you can hold the L for 30 seconds, you may begin training towards a V by gradually working your legs closer to your torso. Think about moving your hips forward (not just your legs) to facilitate this move.

Skinning the Cat:

Start by hanging from a bar with an overhand grip, then begin raising your legs with your knees bent. When your knees are all the way up to your chest, continue to roll your body around to the other side, keeping your legs tucked tight so they don't hit the bar as you pass through. Then fully extend your body while trying to reach your toes toward the ground. This will give you a deep stretch in your shoulders, which is an added benefit of the exercise. Briefly hold the stretch, then slowly reverse your position.

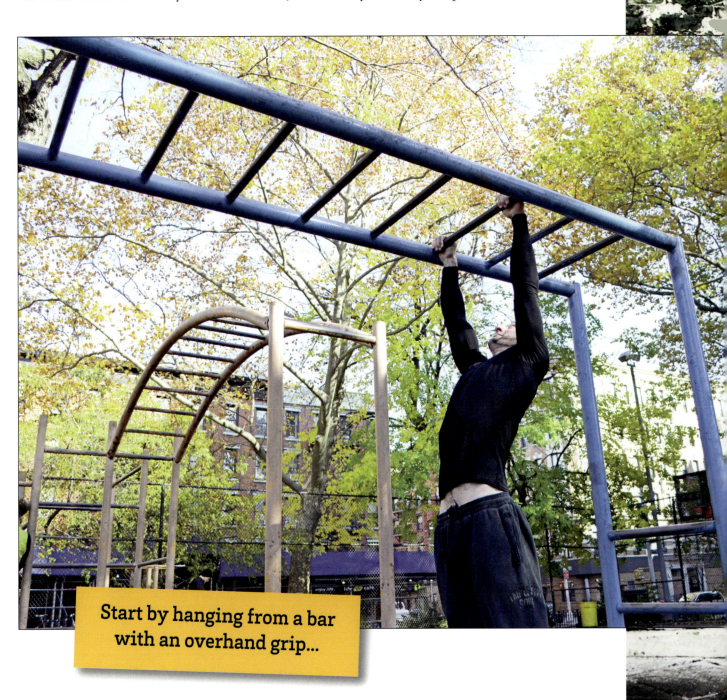

Start by hanging from a bar with an overhand grip...

Skinning the Cat

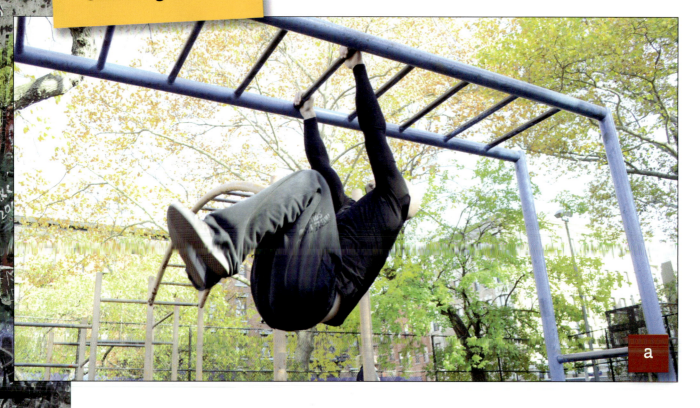

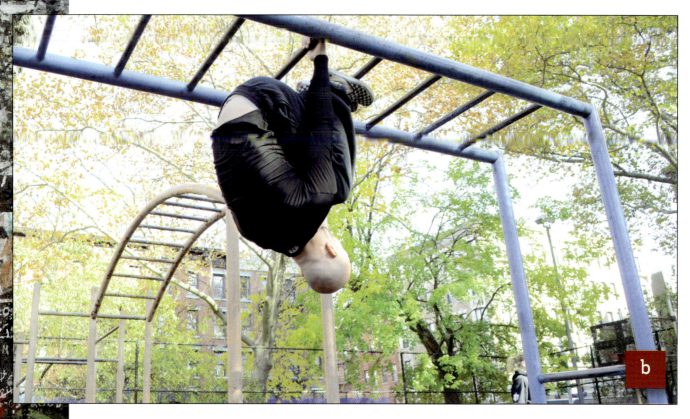

Raising the Bar

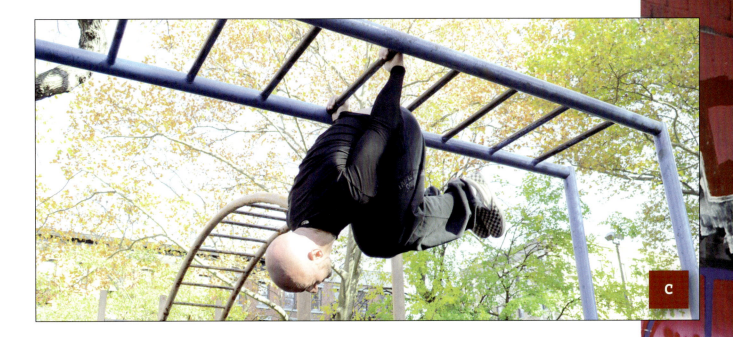

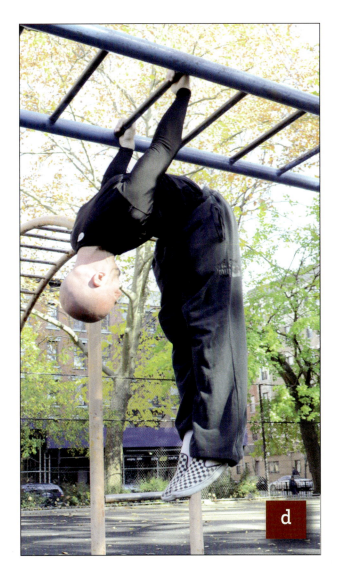

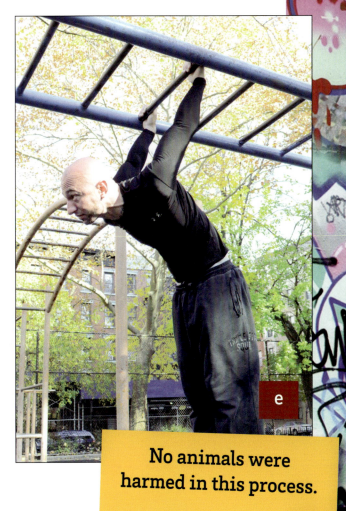

No animals were harmed in this process.

Rollover

A rollover begins almost like a hanging leg raise but continues until your entire body rolls over on top of the bar, leaving you in the same position you'd find yourself in at the top of a muscle-up. To perform a rollover, pull with your arms as you bring your legs up as high as possible, eventually tossing them over the bar. You should feel your center of gravity shift to the opposite side. From here lift your torso, straighten your arms and prepare to drop into another rep. Typically some kipping is involved when performing rollovers, though exceptionally strong individuals can perform the movement slowly. (More on kipping and muscle-ups in the Chapter Five.)

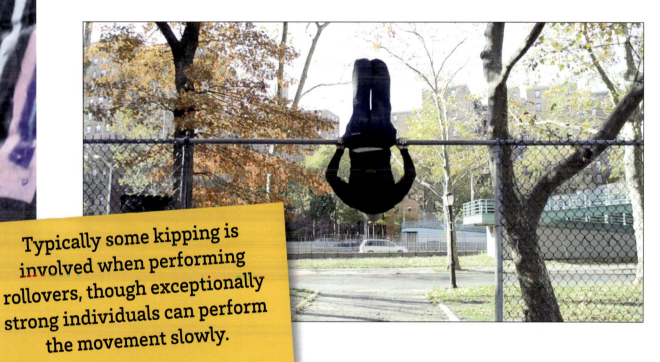

> Typically some kipping is involved when performing rollovers, though exceptionally strong individuals can perform the movement slowly.

One Arm Hanging Leg Raise

The single arm variation of the hanging leg raise isn't just one of the hardest abs exercises, it's actually one of the hardest exercises in all of bar calisthenics. It's honestly unfair to even call it an ab exercise since it requires tremendous grip and shoulder strength as well. Needless to say, it would be foolish to try this one before you get very comfortable with the two arm version. You'll also need to practice hanging from one arm for a while first.

Raising the Bar

Once you can perform ten controlled reps of two arm hanging leg raises and hold yourself for at least 30 seconds from one arm, you might be able to do one or two single arm hanging leg raises. From there you can do several sets of just a couple reps at a time and eventually work your way up. You'll have to go very slowly to avoid swinging around and spinning out of control when you perform this move. Remember to squeeze the bar tight and use the muscles of your back and shoulders to stabilize your body. Anyone who can perform ten reps of this exercise on each side is truly a master of their bodyweight.

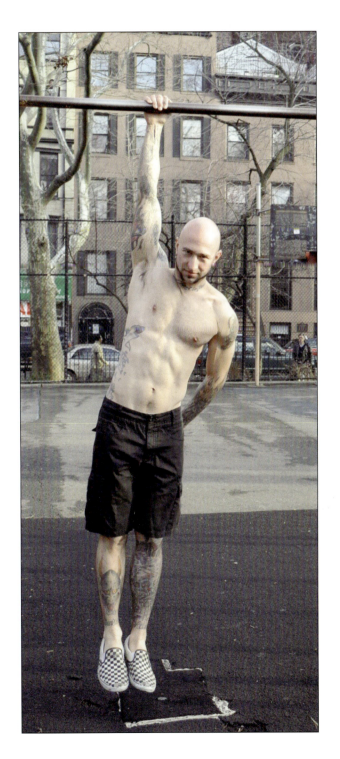
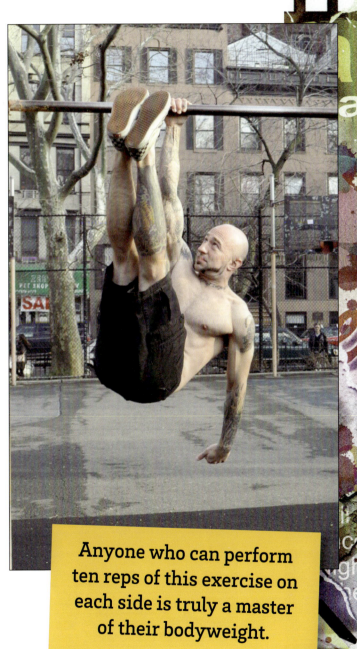

Anyone who can perform ten reps of this exercise on each side is truly a master of their bodyweight.

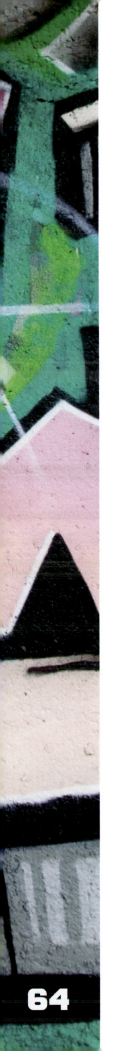

Raising the Bar

Anatomy of a Six Pack

There is a lot more benefit to a strong core than just getting a six-pack, but of course aesthetics is a nice benefit of strength training. Just be careful not to get too carried away with it. While everyone is capable of achieving a flat, toned stomach, not everyone can have a perfect six pack.

The rectus abdominis is one muscle that runs from the sternum to the pelvis, but due to it's ridged shape it can give the illusion of looking like six (or sometimes eight) different muscles. Some ridges in some people's rectus abdominis form even cube shapes while some of us have more crooked looking abs. Even though the basic anatomy is the same, we all have slightly different looking muscles. It's just like how we all have a mouth, a nose and two eyes, yet every person has a unique looking face.

In fact, the same is true for all your muscles - some people's biceps have a nice peak and some don't. Some guys might have a flat-looking chest, others might have a hard time building large shoulders. Different bodies are just shaped differently. Though individual genetics play a part in how your muscles look, nobody is genetically incapable of being lean and muscular. I work hard to make the best of what I got. Do likewise and you might just come close to reaching your full potential. It's actually very simple - but that doesn't mean it's easy.

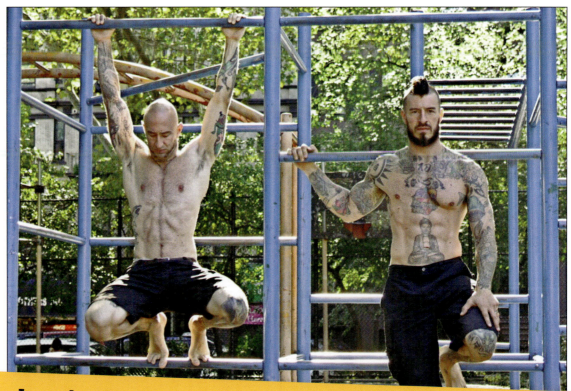

It used to drive me nuts that Danny's abs are more symmetrical than mine, but I guess mine ain't so bad either.

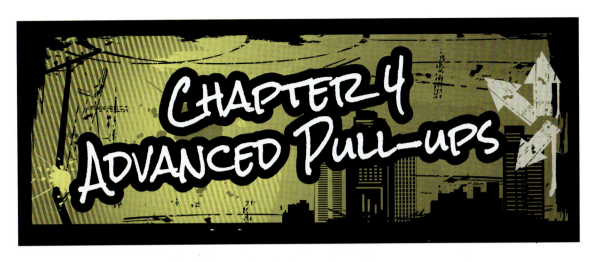

Chapter 4
Advanced Pull-ups

"Hear me now and believe me later..."
–Hans and Franz

When I was starting out in the fitness industry, I took personal training classes and read lots of textbooks so I could learn all the best workouts and newest innovations. I saw a lot in the literature about lat pull-down machines, but not all that much about the trusted pull-up. The few things I did encounter in praise of this glorious exercise still stressed one particular caution. The experts all seemed to agree that one should never go behind the neck on a pull-up (or even on a pull-down machine, for that matter). If you ask me, though, that's a load of bullshit.

A lot of the fitness industry has questionable motives, but generally most fitness advice is given with safety in mind. This is a big part of why mainstream fitness tends to shy away from pull-ups in general. The average person might be too weak and/or out of touch with their body to attempt a pull-up without hurting themselves, but hopefully if you managed to get your hands on this book you won't have to worry about that.

Sure, you could potentially hurt your shoulders if you do behind the neck pull-ups before you are strong enough (or flexible enough). You could also get hurt behind the wheel of a car if you don't know how to drive. That doesn't mean cars are bad.

The behind the neck pull-up is an advanced variation (that's why it's in this chapter), so make sure you can do at least ten clean overhand pull-ups before you embark on any of the exercises discussed here. It can be tempting to jump ahead in your training, but keep in mind that your body is only as strong as its weakest link. Even the great Achilles was taken down by a single arrow. Honor your body and it will honor you.

Behind the Neck

In addition to serious upper-back strength, safely performing a behind the neck pull-up requires better than average shoulder flexibility. If you feel pain when doing this or any other exercise, you should stop or it's your own damn fault if you get hurt. It's also never a good idea to shrug your shoulders up when doing pull-ups, but it's especially true in the case of the behind the neck variation.

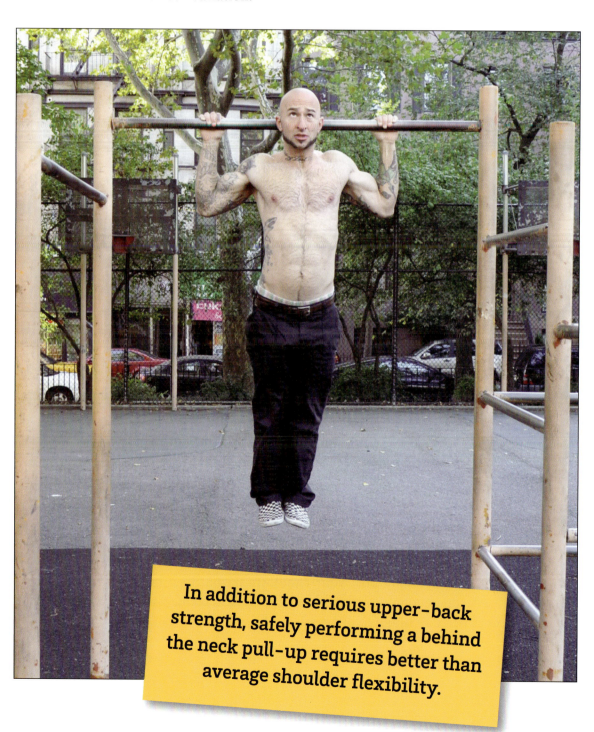

> In addition to serious upper-back strength, safely performing a behind the neck pull-up requires better than average shoulder flexibility.

Get "Width" It

The standard pull-up grip is just outside of shoulder width. Anything wider or narrower will make the exercise more challenging. In general, shifting your grip to a wider position will add more emphasis on your lats and other upper back muscles, while going narrow will work your forearms and biceps a bit harder. The difference is subtle, however, and any type of pull-up works every muscle in your upper body to some degree. It's great to practice getting comfortable with all the different grips and eventually the disparity of difficulty between grips will begin to even out.

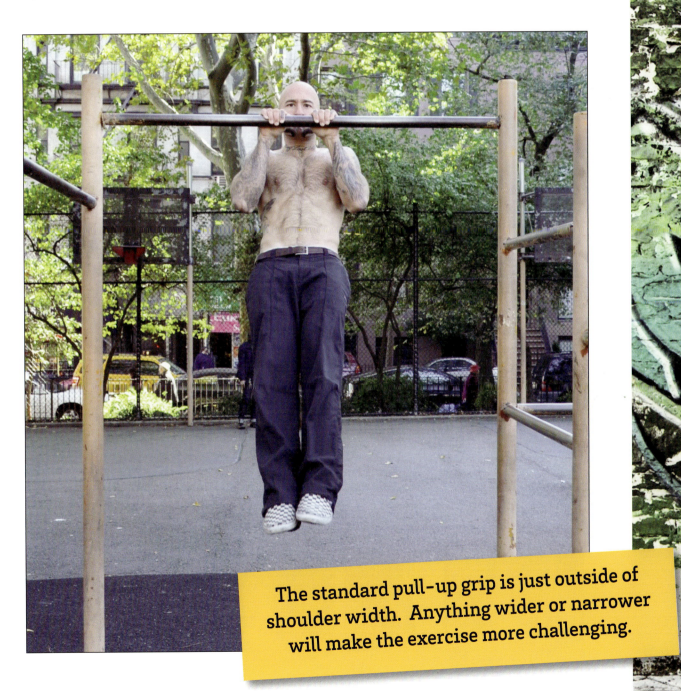

The standard pull-up grip is just outside of shoulder width. Anything wider or narrower will make the exercise more challenging.

Mixed Grip

A mixed grip pull-up is done with one hand supinated and one hand pronated. This variation can make for an interesting stability challenge as you try to keep your torso facing forward. It can also be a useful tool for beginners who may be having a hard time transitioning from chin-ups to pull-ups.

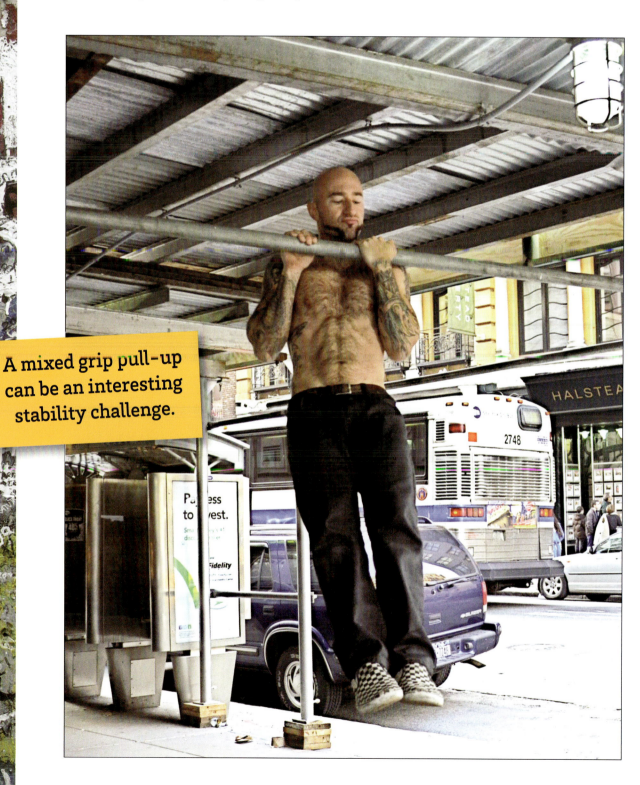

A mixed grip pull-up can be an interesting stability challenge.

Headbanger pull-up

Whether you're a fan of heavy metal music or not, this is a fun and worthwhile exercise. The headbanger pull-up begins with your chin just below the bar. From here the objective is to extend your upper body away from the bar while reaching your legs out to counterbalance, then return to the start position and repeat. Almost like a bodyweight biceps curl, the headbanger pull-up is also a great core exercise.

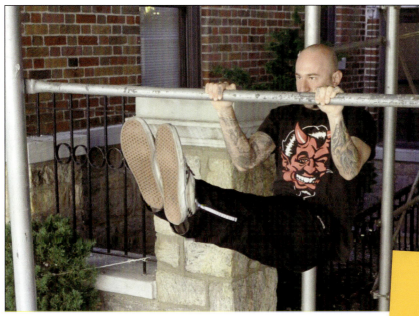

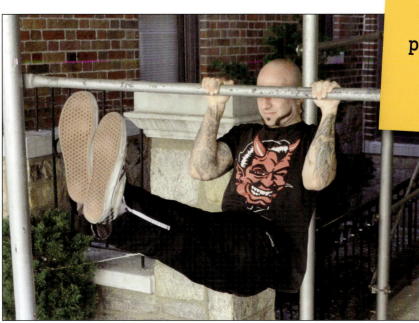

> Almost like a bodyweight biceps curl, the headbanger pull-up is also a great core exercise.

Going Commando

The commando pull-up is another great variation to have in your arsenal. A commando pull-up is similar to a mixed grip pull-up, except you use a narrow grip and pull your head to the side of the bar, alternating which side with each rep. If you aren't strong enough for this yet, you can try a modified version with your feet up on a nearby bar or other object.

It's good to practice switching the position of your hands on alternating sets with variations like mixed grip and commando pull-ups. For example, if my right hand is closer to my face on the first set, I'll keep my left hand closer on set number two. For this reason, I typically will do an even number of sets if I'm using these pull-up variations in my regimen.

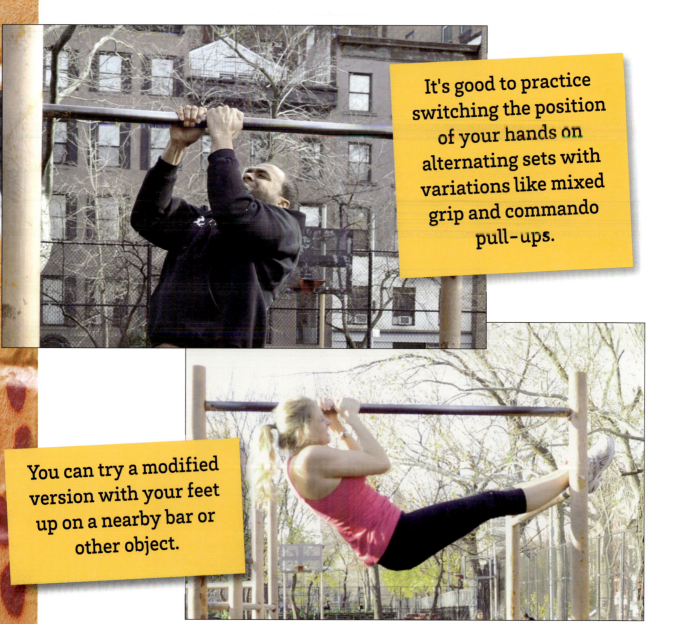

It's good to practice switching the position of your hands on alternating sets with variations like mixed grip and commando pull-ups.

You can try a modified version with your feet up on a nearby bar or other object.

Archer Pull-up

An archer pull-up involves keeping one arm straight while pulling your body towards your opposite hand. The top position resembles that of someone drawing a bow and arrow. When performing the archer pull-up as practice for the one arm pull-up, try to do as much of the work as possible with the arm closer to you. Think of your extended arm simply as a means of giving yourself assistance. Use it as little as possible. Eventually you won't need it at all. (More on one arm pull-ups in Chapter 8).

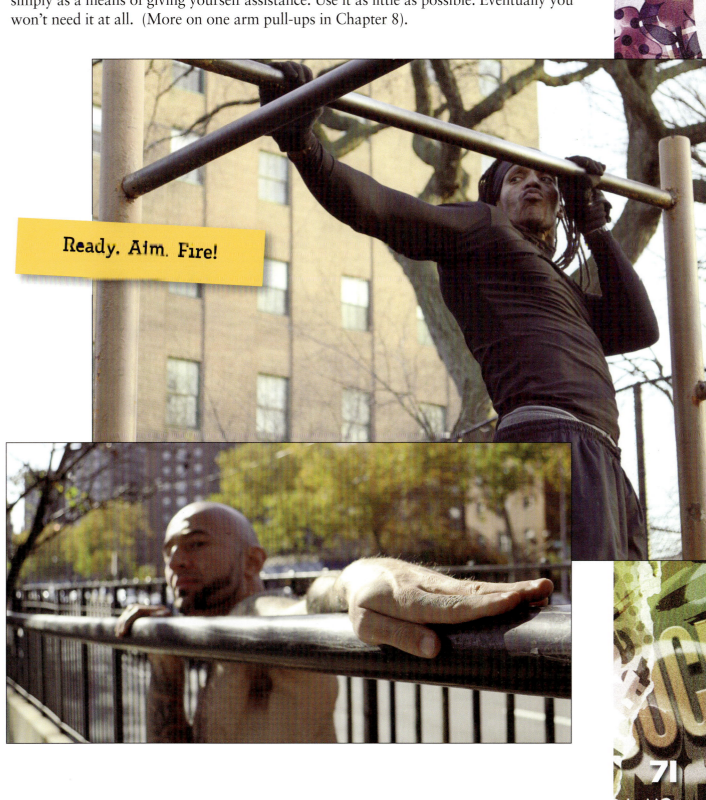

Ready. Aim. Fire!

Typewriters

Once you get to the top position of the archer pull-up, you may decide to perform a typewriter. This is another exercise whose name is a literal description of the movement pattern. Just like an old-school typewriter resetting at the end of a line, when you perform this move your chin stays above the bar as you slide your body towards the opposite side. The typewriter demands strong shoulders and a powerful core. It's harder than it might look!

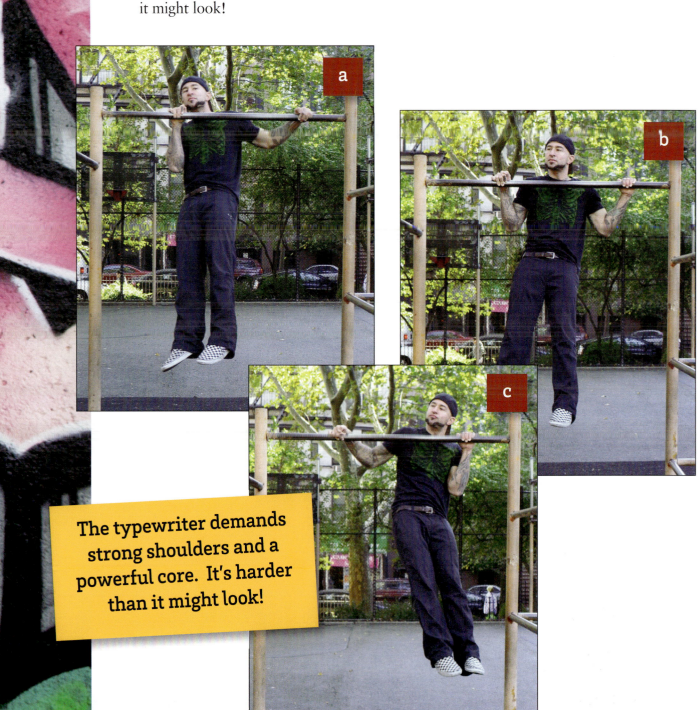

> The typewriter demands strong shoulders and a powerful core. It's harder than it might look!

X Pull-up

As the name implies, the X pull-up involves crossing your arms over each other into a letter X formation. This can either be done on one straight bar or two parallel bars. Each version offers their own specific challenges, though the rotational pull of your arms is a factor for either one. You'll have to go slowly on the way up to keep your body from spinning around. Be careful with your shoulders here, as some flexibility is required to properly perform the X pull-up. You may also be surprised by how much grip and forearm strength is needed to perform this one.

Though it's a cool looking move and something you may find worth trying, I've never seen the X pull-up as an essential variation. For the love of pull-ups, I'm including it here, but the others on this list will likely be more worth your while.

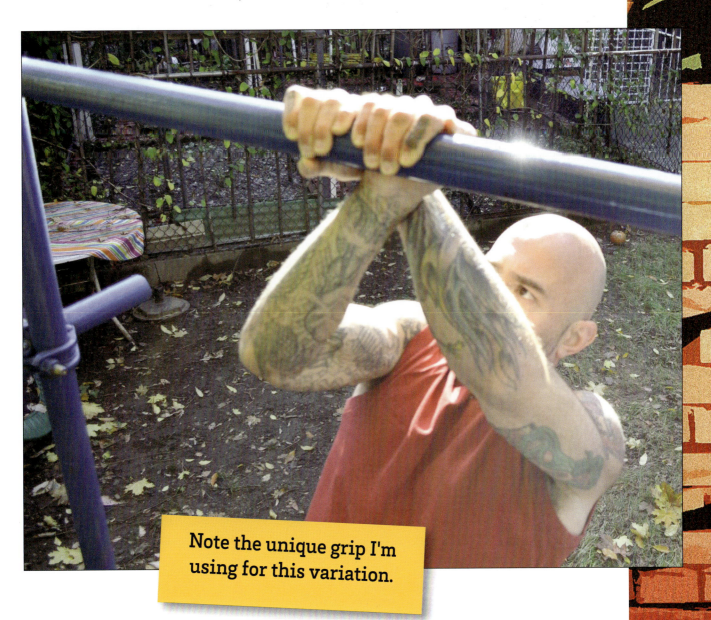

Note the unique grip I'm using for this variation.

RAISING THE BAR

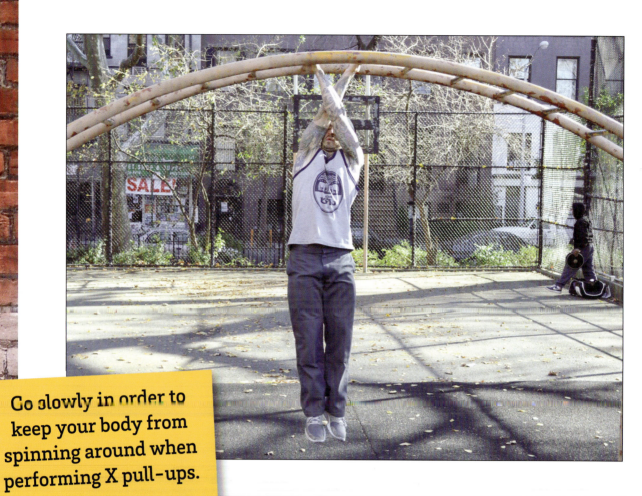

Go slowly in order to keep your body from spinning around when performing X pull-ups.

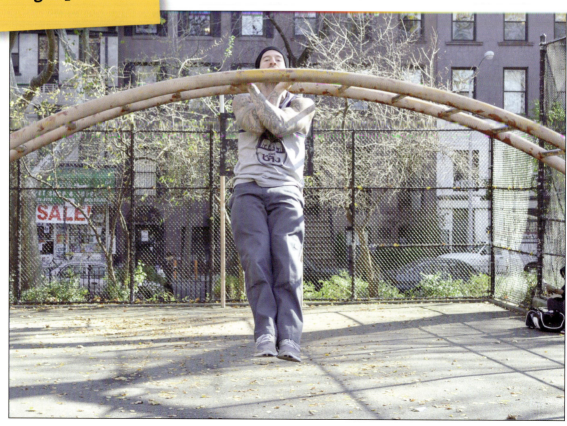

Decline Australian Pull-up

As I mentioned in chapter one, the Australian pull-up is a great technique for beginners to use while building towards full pull-ups, but the Australian is still a worthwhile tool for someone of any strength level. Remember that the Australian pull-up is really more of a row than a pull-up, so it's worth keeping in your repertoire in some capacity as it's almost an entirely different exercise.

While a beginner should start with a bar that's around waist height, when you've advanced beyond that you should use a lower bar to decrease your leverage. Eventually you'll need to put your feet up on a second bar to put your body on a declined angle in order to make this exercise challenging enough. You can also experiment with plyometric Australian pull-ups by explosively switching from an overhand to underhand grip in between reps, or sliding your hands from a wide grip to a narrow grip and back. There is always a way to add a new challenge to a basic exercise.

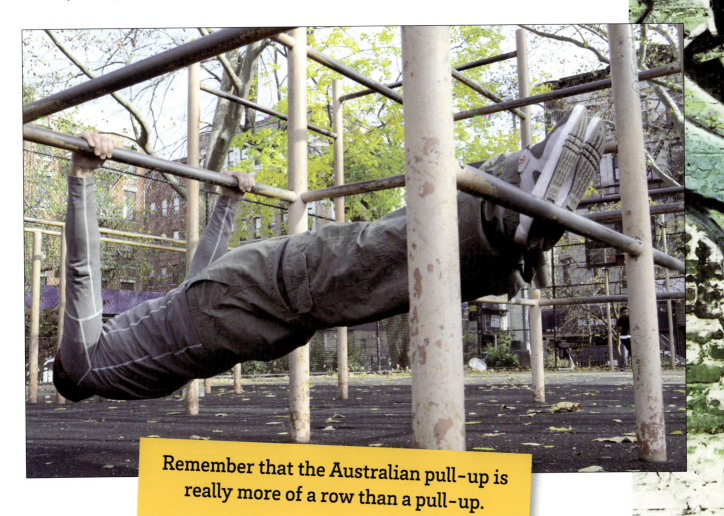

Remember that the Australian pull-up is really more of a row than a pull-up.

L-sit Pull-up

Keeping your legs at a 90 degree angle to your body while performing pull-ups adds a tremendous amount of difficulty. Your abs will have to work very hard to maintain the position as you pull your chin past the bar. Additionally, the balance changes through the range of motion during an L-sit pull-up, forcing you to slow down in order to maintain control.

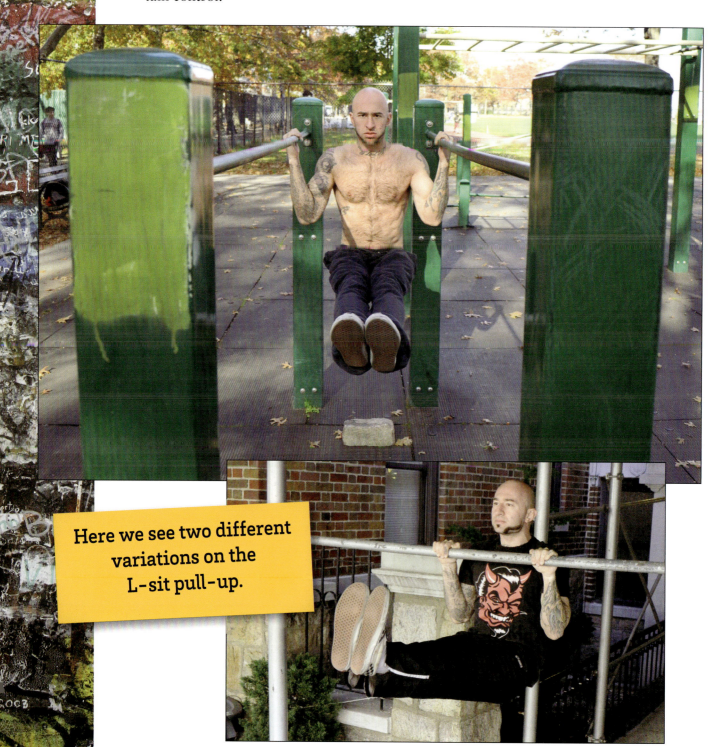

Here we see two different variations on the L-sit pull-up.

Kipping is Appreciated

In the world of pull-ups, kipping (using the momentum of your hips to generate power) is a highly contested topic. Some say that kipping is cheating, but I think that's a narrow-minded view. While a kipping pull-up won't help you build strength as directly as strict form pull-ups, learning to kip can still be a useful skill. Even if you're already proficient at standard pull-ups, working on your kip can help you on your way towards plyo pull-ups and muscle-ups.

As kipping pull-ups require less upper body strength than standard pull-ups, people might consider kipping to be a beginner technique. Yet here I am writing about it in the advanced pull-ups section. That's because I think everyone who considers themselves advanced in the world of pull-ups should be able to kip. I've seen a lot of people who were strong on pull-ups but struggled with learning the muscle-up because they couldn't figure out the kip. I was once one of those people myself!

While pull-ups are typically performed by going straight up and down, the kipping pull-up creates an arc, rather than a straight line, as a means to quickly propel the body upward.

To train your kip, start by hanging on the bar with your shoulders pulled down into their sockets. Swing your legs and use your hips to generate momentum. Remember playing on the swings in the playground when you were a little kid?

Swing your hips and push your chest forward to get some momentum.

Raising the Bar

When you get the feel for this, you will soon be able to generate upward momentum by whipping your body to create an S shape movement pattern on the way up. When your legs are in front of your body at the end of your swing, push your chest forward and let your back arch slightly, this will generate more return force on the way back. Think about what happens to a rubber band when you stretch it out and then let it go. When you kip, you are trying to use your body like a rubber band, so make it snappy!

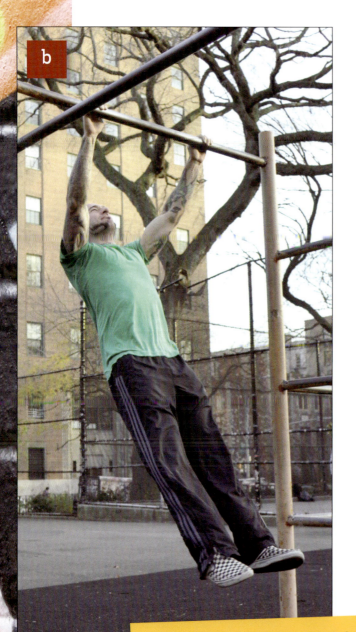
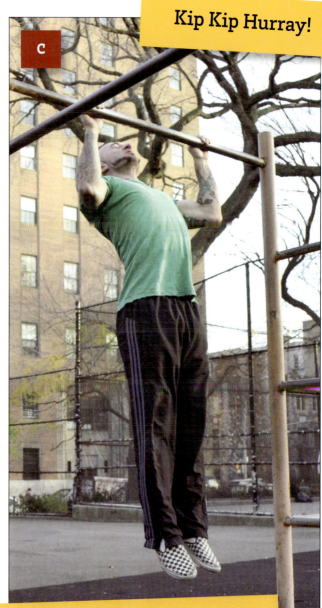

Kip Kip Hurray!

When you get the feel for this, you will soon be able to generate upward momentum by whipping your body to create an S shape movement pattern on the way up.

Plyo pull-ups

Once you've gotten confident with controlled pull-ups and you've learned how to kip, you can put the two together and begin training plyo-pull-ups. Any type of explosive pull-up in which you let go of the bar is a plyo. When you perform plyo pull-ups, think about pulling your chin over the bar as fast and explosively as possible. In fact, don't think of pulling your chin over the bar - think of pulling the bar below your chest! Once you get the feel for this, try opening your hands for a split second. Eventually you can develop enough power to take your hands off long enough to clap. Maybe even behind your back.

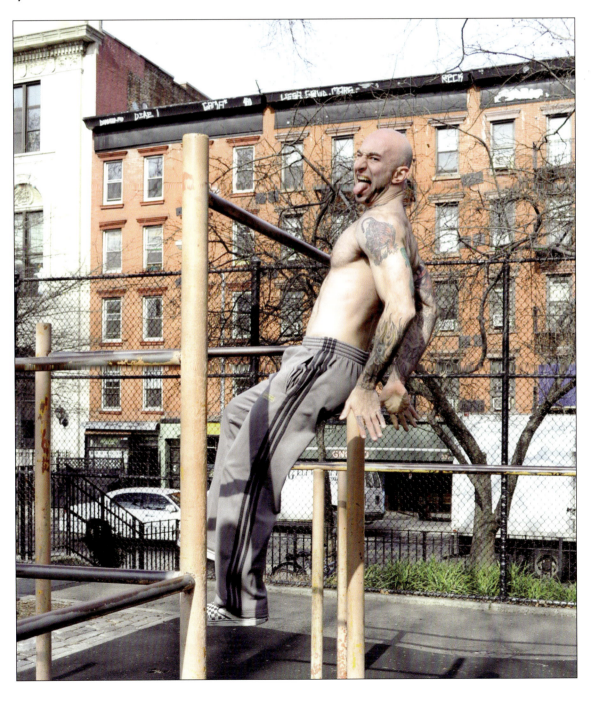

There are lots of other variations on the plyo pull-up. You can switch from an overhand to an underhand grip, slide from a narrow grip to a wide grip, try to touch your toes in mid-air or anything else you can think of. Once you develop the strength, power and confidence to go for harder moves, you can improvise challenging freestyle workouts in just about any setting.

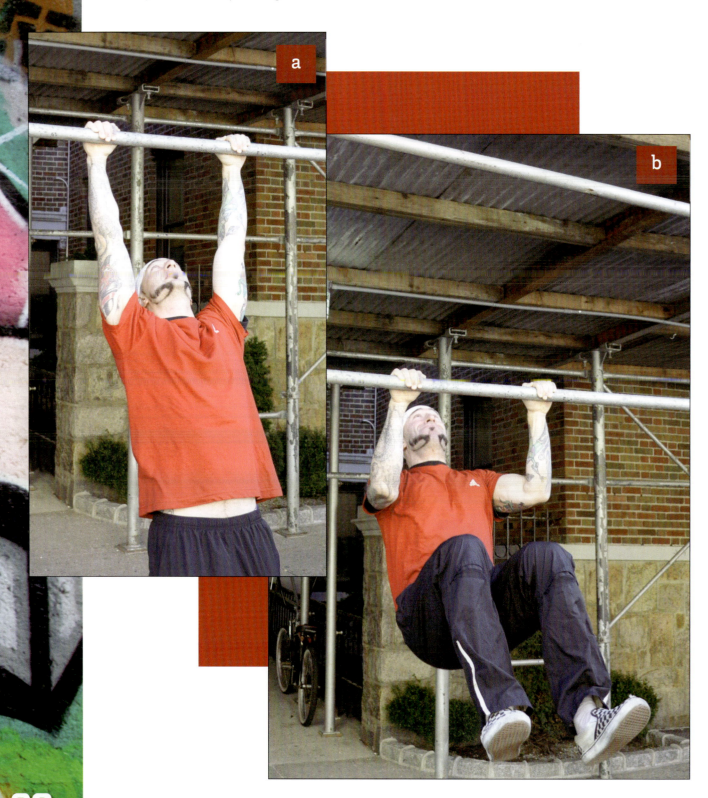

Raising the Bar

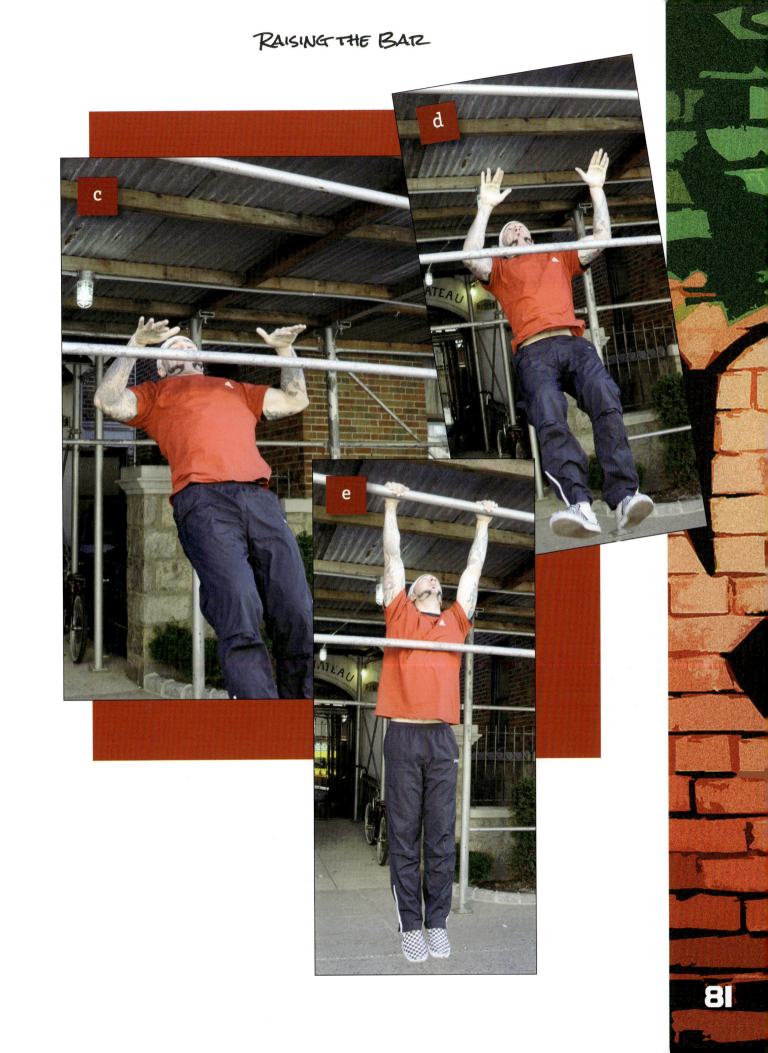

Do Your Thing

In the world of pull-ups there is plenty of room for personal style and creativity. No matter how many pull-ups you see, you'll never see them all. Pull-ups are like fingerprints, every individual has a distinctive way of doing their thing on the bar. The endless possibilities of bar training is the beauty of it all.

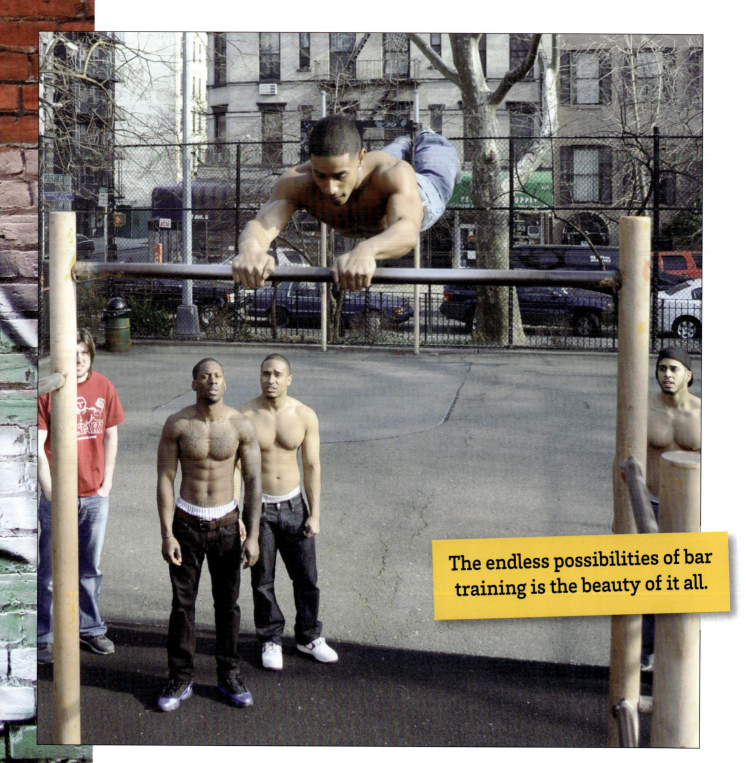

The endless possibilities of bar training is the beauty of it all.

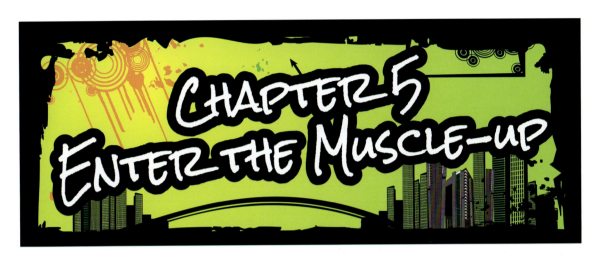

Chapter 5: Enter the Muscle-up

"He who makes a beast of himself gets rid of the pain of being a man."
–Samuel Johnson

Though the muscle-up is most commonly known as a gymnastics exercise, it is also one of the most intense calisthenics moves out there. Gymnasts don't actually get points for muscle-ups, but they must do one in order to get in position to begin their routine. That's right - for a gymnast, a muscle-up isn't even a real move! That's not a statement against the muscle-up, however. It is a testament to the level of elite gymnastic competitions. After all, a gymnast would look pretty silly if they just started busting out pull-ups during their routine, but that doesn't mean the pull-up ain't an amazing exercise!

Muscle...almost

The first time I tried to do a muscle-up, I was already quite good at pull-ups, so I expected to be able to do it right away. Needless to say, it didn't happen quite that easily. Like anyone else, I had to practice a lot to get the timing right. Getting a feel for the movement pattern takes practice, even if you're already strong. The muscle-up is a very unique skill that can single-handedly build serious strength and sculpt a powerful upper body. The only catch is that you already have to be strong in order to do that first one.

No other exercise requires both pulling and pushing power quite like the muscle-up, but it is also one of the most demanding abs exercises as well. You get a lot of bang for your buck with this one. The muscle-up is truly the ultimate upper body exercise.

Raising the Bar

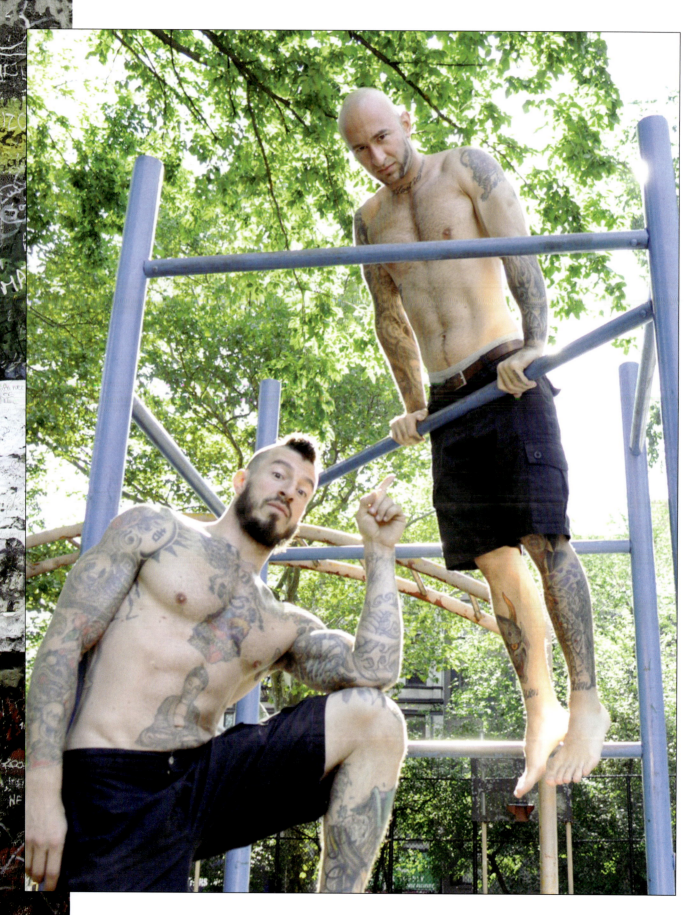

Raising the Bar

In the beginning of this book I told you the only bar exercises were pull-ups, dips and hanging leg raises, and everything else is just a variation or combination of those things. Some people mistakenly think the muscle-up is just a combination of a pull-up and a dip, but in reality a muscle-up is closer to being a combination of all three. The pull-up and dip part should be obvious, but you must also squeeze your abs tight and move your legs away from your body to get around the bar, just like when performing a hanging leg raise.

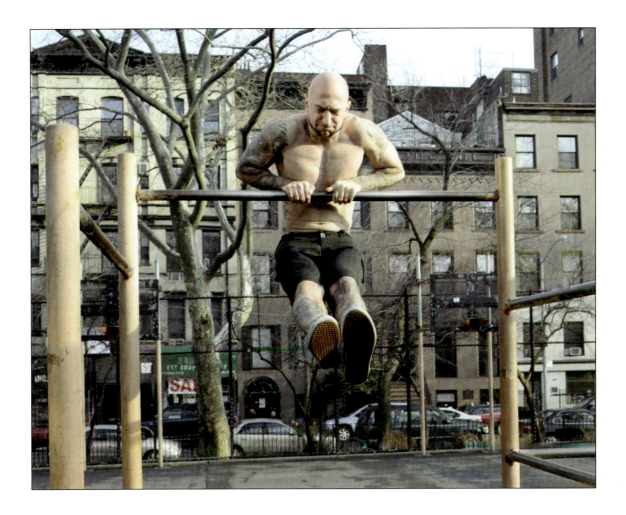

To practice muscle-ups, you'll need a bar with plenty of overhead clearance. Ironically, many high-tech gyms lack a simple straight bar. Watch out for universal machines with all those fancy ergonomic handles - they're lousy for muscle-up training. You're probably better off not going to a gym anyway. It shouldn't be too hard to find a local park with a suitable bar. After all, when was the last time you saw someone do a muscle-up at a gym?

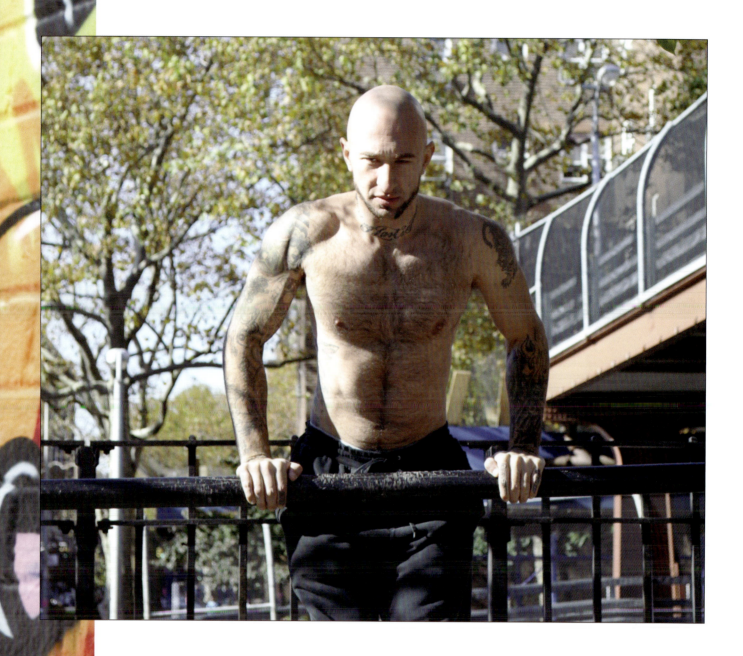

Beyond Pull-ups

When you do a muscle-up, instead of simply trying to pull your chin past the bar, the objective is to pull (and then push) your entire upper body up and over. If you've never done this move before, get ready for a humbling. Even if you can do lots of pull-ups and dips, you'll still need some practice on the transition before you will be able to execute a proper muscle-up.

As I mentioned in chapter four, kipping pull-ups and plyo-pull-ups are a fantastic precursor to the muscle-up. It can also be helpful to practice explosive pull-ups with an exaggerated range of motion. Instead of stopping when the bar is below your chin, pull that sucker all the way down past your chest. Get as far over the bar as you can!

Though there is no set rule for how many reps are needed as a prerequisite, I recommend getting well into double digits on both pull-ups and straight bar dips before attempting the muscle-up. But remember that proficiency in these moves doesn't guarantee you success. While some people who can only manage six or seven pull-ups can muster up a muscle-up, others who can bang out twenty dead hang pull-ups still continually fail at getting through the sticking point. The muscle-up is a unique challenge and must be treated as such.

When starting out, it can be helpful to practice a modified muscle-up on a bar that is about chest height so you can use your legs to help jump into it. (If you can't find a low bar, bring a step or a bench up to a high bar.) This will let you get a feel for the transition from being under the bar to getting on top without having to overcome the resistance of your full bodyweight. With practice, you'll learn to rely on your legs less and do most of the work with your upper body.

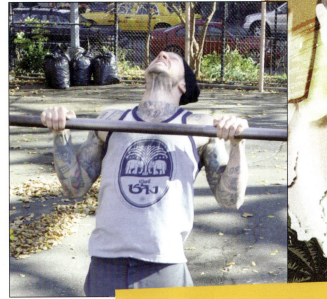

Get as far over the bar as you can!

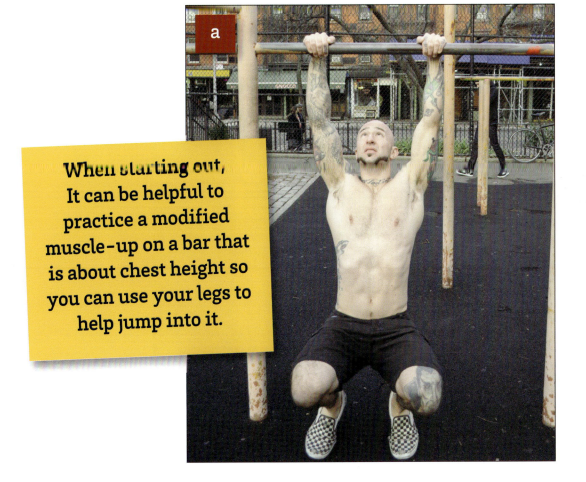

When starting out, it can be helpful to practice a modified muscle-up on a bar that is about chest height so you can use your legs to help jump into it.

Raising the Bar

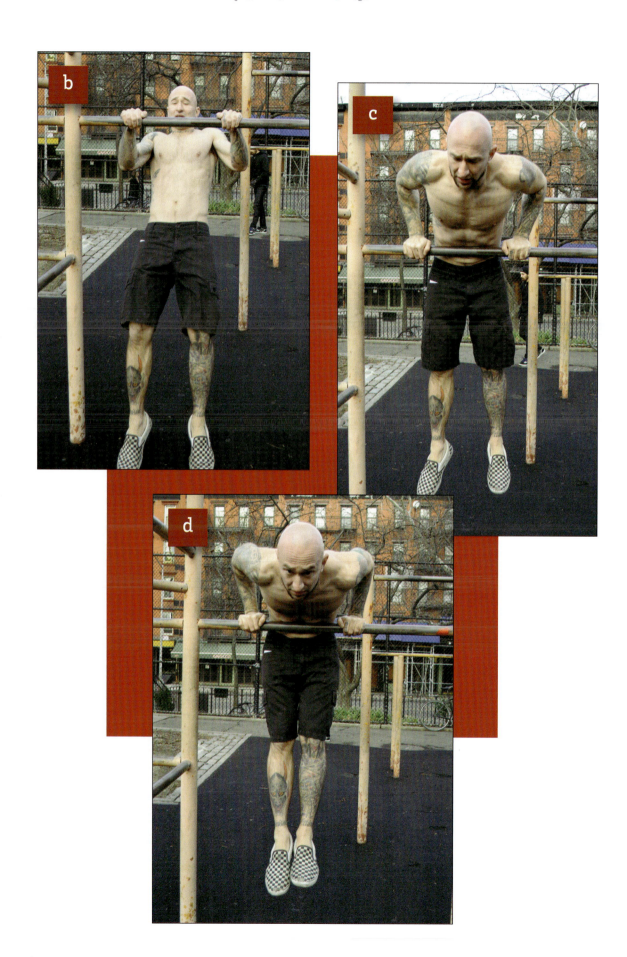

The False Grip

Some people will find it helpful to use a false grip when performing a muscle-up on a bar. The false grip in an exaggerated hook grip that entails bending your wrists over the bar so that your palms are facing down toward the ground. The false grip can allow for an easier transition between the pull-up and dip phases of the muscle-up.

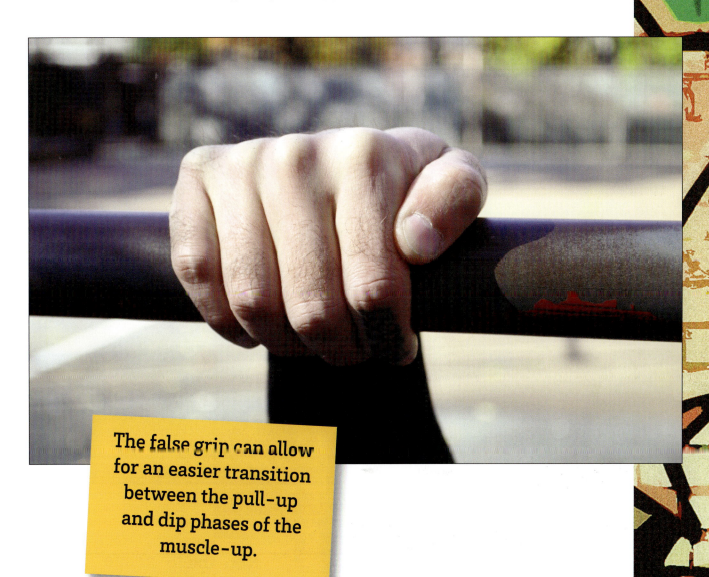

The false grip can allow for an easier transition between the pull-up and dip phases of the muscle-up.

Be Negative

Just like when you are working on getting your first pull-up, it can be helpful to practice negatives and use manual assistance while learning to do a muscle-up. If you are going to spot someone on a muscle-up, I suggest giving them a boost by holding them under one or both heels, as if you were helping them over a fence.

Another technique that can be helpful when starting out is to practice from the top down. Perform a rollover (or find some other way to get to the top of the muscle-up position), then try to create momentum by dropping down. Use that downward momentum to propel yourself back up into your muscle-up. Imagine that your body is a rubber band being stretched out. Remember what happens to that rubber band when you stretch it out and then let it go.

Speaking of which, remember that "S" shape we talked about for kipping pull-ups? When you perform a muscle-up, you will again need to utilize the S-shape movement as your body moves around the bar. You do not go up in a straight line.

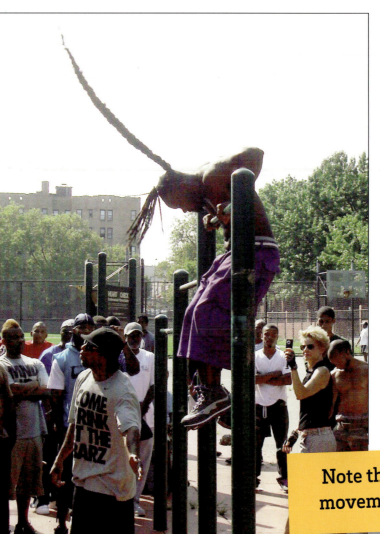

Since the range of motion for a muscle-up is much larger than that of a pull-up, you are going to have to do a larger "S" to get yourself over the bar. Exaggerating this "S" shape can allow you to get better leverage and momentum, so use it to your advantage, especially when learning the movement pattern.

Note the "S" shape movement pattern.

Raising the Bar

No one's first muscle-up looks great. In the beginning you'll probably need to squirm your way through the sticking point and you'll likely wind up with one arm going over the bar before the other. It's also common for beginners to bend their knees and kick a lot from the legs. While this is not ideal, it is okay as long as you don't let it become a habit. Once you can do a few reps, work on cleaning up your form. Eventually you should be able to do muscle-ups with your legs straight and minimal hip movement. There is always more room for growth in your training.

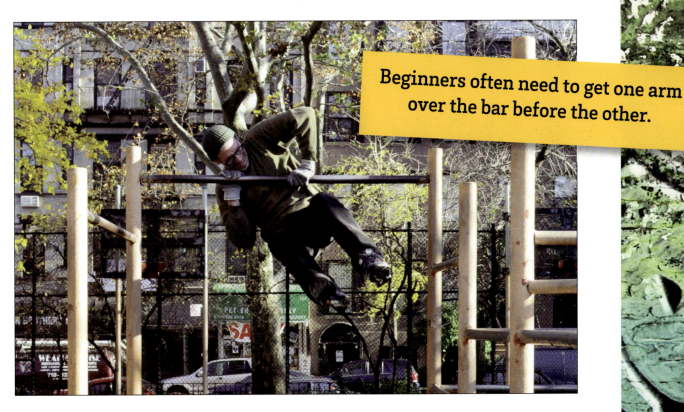

Beginners often need to get one arm over the bar before the other.

Muscle-up Variations

Though it may take you weeks, months or possibly longer to get your first decent muscle-up, once you get comfortable with muscle-ups, you will eventually be ready to move onto harder variations.

Close grip and wide grip muscle-up

Just like pull-ups, muscle-ups are typically done with the hands just outside shoulder width, but they can also be done wider or narrower for an extra challenge. The close-grip muscle-up is a particularly challenging move. Work on gradually bringing your hands closer together over time, eventually building to the point where they are touching.

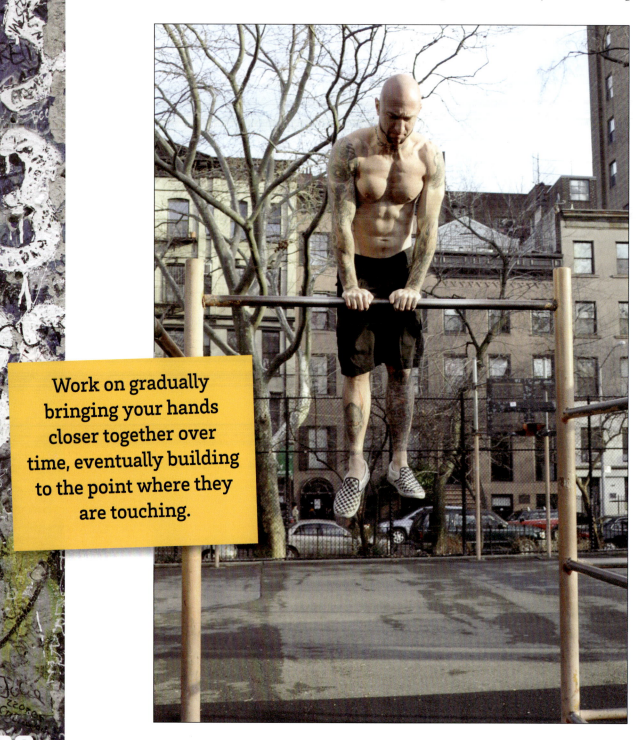

Work on gradually bringing your hands closer together over time, eventually building to the point where they are touching.

Slow muscle-up

Once you've gotten a feel for kipping into a muscle-up, performing a slow muscle-up is a worthwhile challenge. After you can perform six or seven kipping muscle-ups, you should be ready to go for it.

As I mentioned before, I sometimes use a false grip for muscle-ups, but there's actually a special false grip that I like for *slow* muscle-ups. For this variation I like to have my closed fist resting on top of the bar with the bar in the crook of my wrist. This really cooks my forearms, but it allows for better leverage when aiming to keep the movement slow.

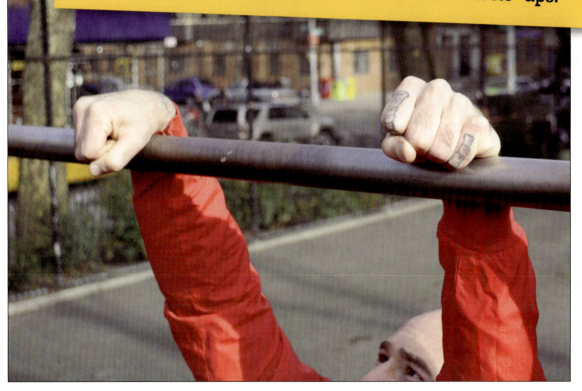

I sometimes use a false grip for muscle-ups, but there's actually a special false grip that I like for slow muscle-ups.

When you do a slow muscle-up, you'll really need to reach your legs away from your body during the transition phase in order to counter balance your weight behind the bar. The carryover from hanging leg raises can make a big difference here but it still takes a lot of practice. It is also another instance in which practicing slow negatives can be helpful.

Raising the Bar

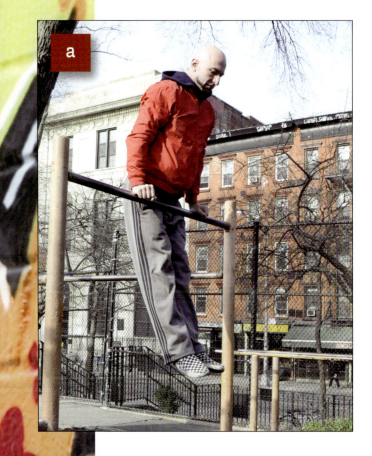
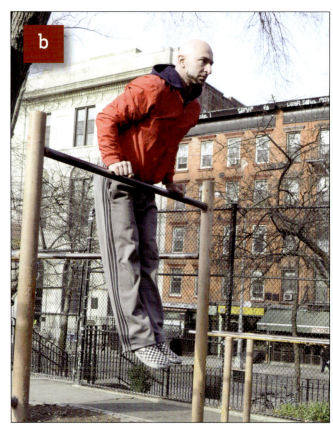
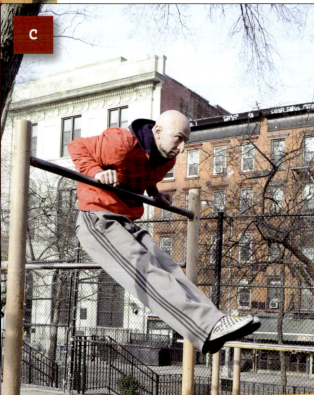
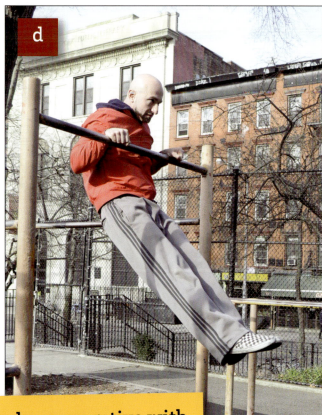

Here we see a slow muscle-up negative with the exaggerated false grip.

Raising the Bar

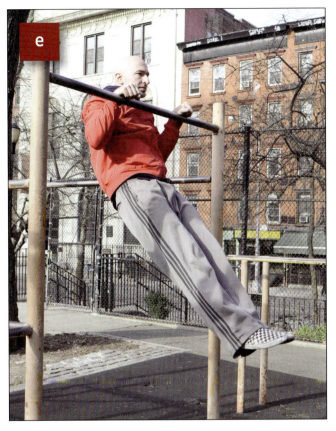
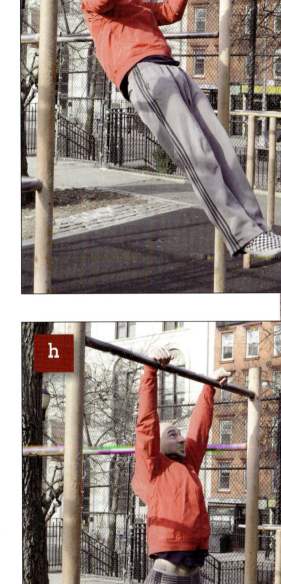
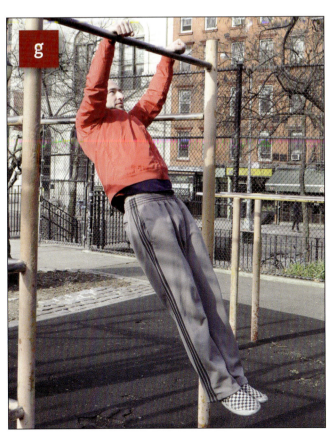

Muscle-up on Parallel Bars

Performing a muscle-up on parallel bars requires monstrous grip strength as well as total body control. If you're going to try this move, get comfortable with a slow muscle-up on the high bar first, then take some time to get a feel for hanging off the end of the parallel bars. You'll have to use a false grip with the end of the bars against your forearms. You'll also need to tuck your legs or do an L-hold to keep your feet off the floor. Those two things alone can require some practice. After that, start working on pull-ups from this position. Soon you'll be ready to muscle-up all the way to the top. When you go for a muscle-up between parallel bars remember that your chest can pitch forward between your hands, almost more like a muscle-up on rings than one on a bar.

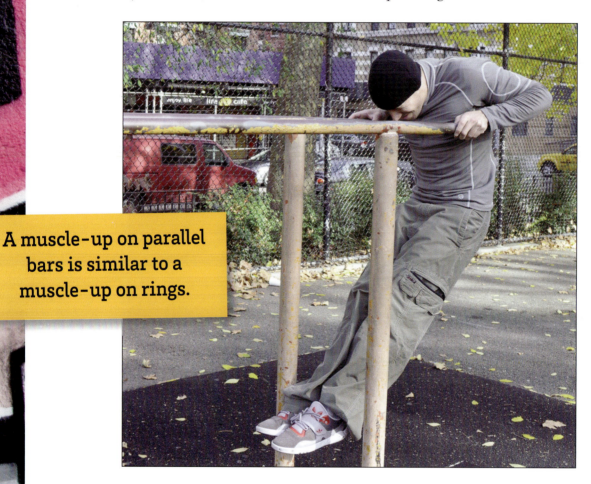

A muscle-up on parallel bars is similar to a muscle-up on rings.

Clap muscle-up

If you do enough muscle-ups, eventually you can try to push beyond the normal range of motion and propel yourself completely off the bar. Once you're in the air, you may choose to toss in a clap or other freestyle movement of your choosing. When practicing plyo muscle-ups, you can use your hips to "cast off" the bar for more height.

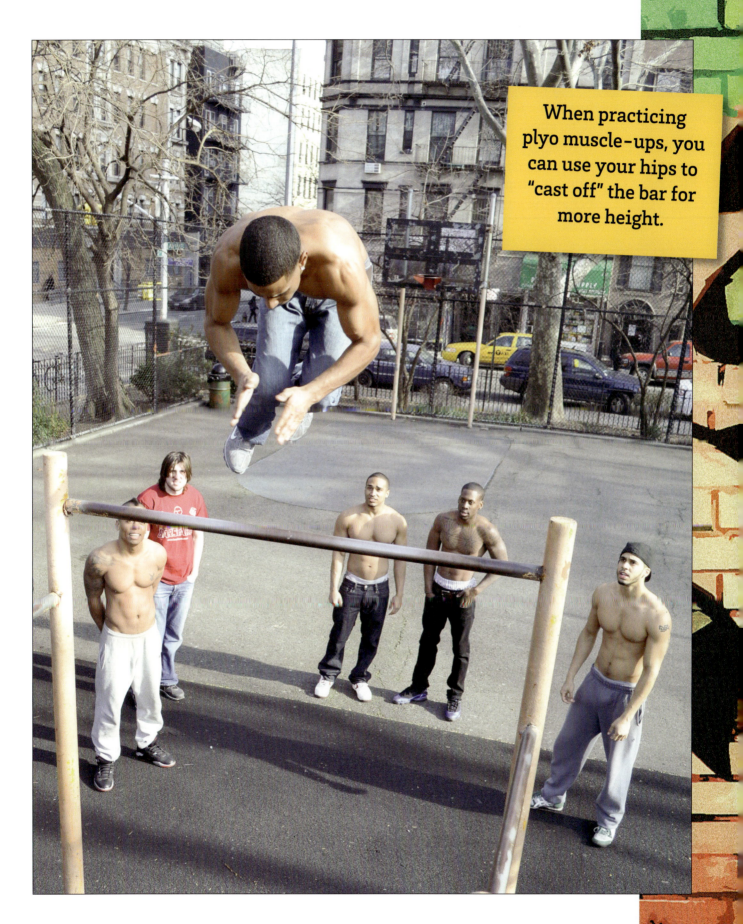

When practicing plyo muscle-ups, you can use your hips to "cast off" the bar for more height.

Muscle-over

A muscle-over takes the plyo muscle-up to the next level. Instead of just getting a little hang time at the top, a muscle-over involves throwing your entire body over the bar. Remember to bounce your hips off the bar to get a little extra momentum. Psychologically, the muscle-over can be quite intimidating at first, but if you really want this move, don't let your fear stop you from trying! If you can do a muscle-up and a vault, you can do a muscle-over. You may find it helpful to rest your outside foot on the bar as you go over to spot yourself as you get more comfortable with the maneuver.

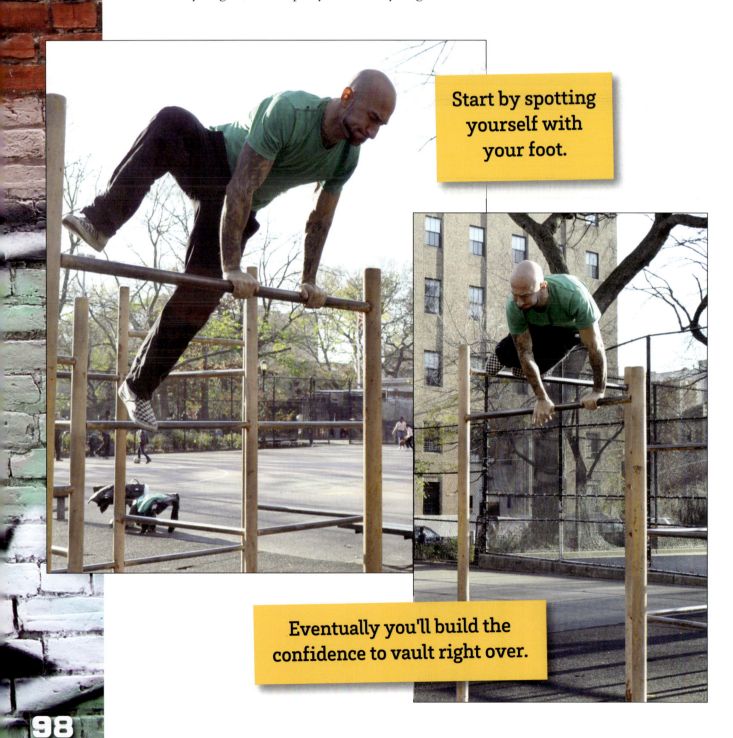

Start by spotting yourself with your foot.

Eventually you'll build the confidence to vault right over.

Standing Muscle-over

This is a variation on the muscle-over than involves landing on top of the bar instead of jumping completely over it. It's a cool looking freestyle move that takes balance and bravery! Try this one at your own risk!

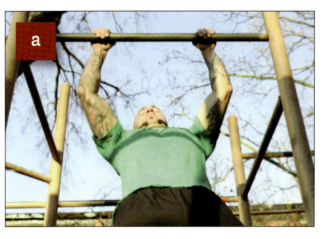

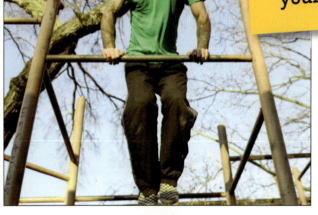

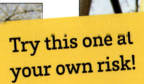

Try this one at your own risk!

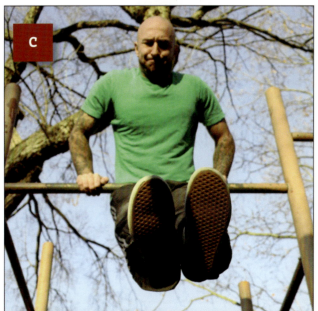

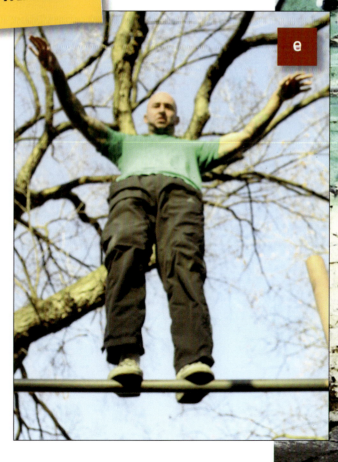

Mixed grip muscle-up

Performing a muscle-up with one hand under and one hand over is harder than it may seem. Creating a smooth transition from under the bar to being on top is quite challenging in this position, as the underhand side will have a hard time rolling over the bar. Consequently, the overhand side needs to do most of the work. At first, you may find yourself wiggling a bit through the transition as you find a way to work your supinated hand over and around. Keep practicing!

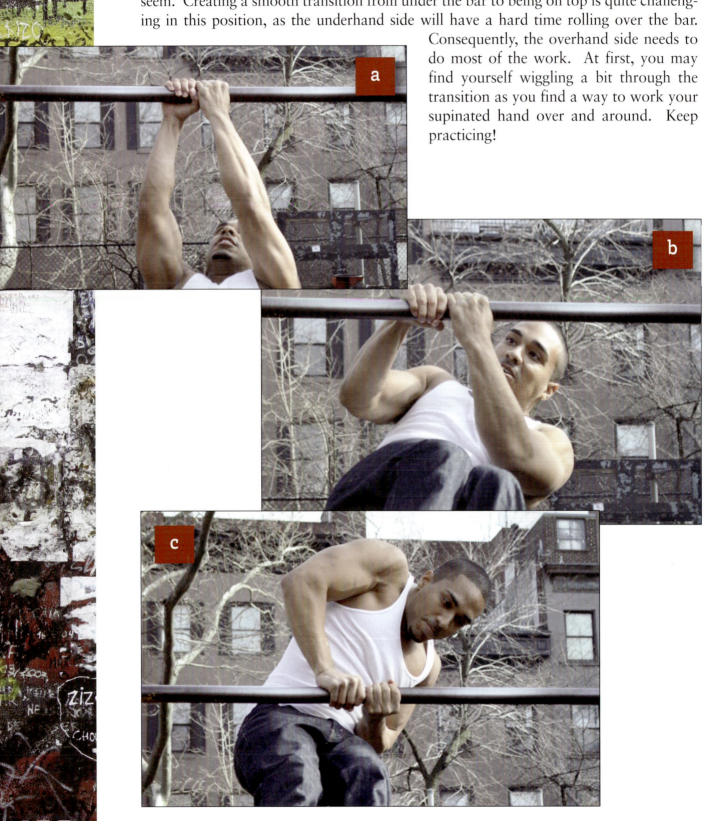

RAISING THE BAR

d

Creating a smooth transition from under the bar to being on top is quite challenging in this position, as the underhand side will have a hard time rolling over the bar.

e

101

Reverse Grip Muscle-up

Unlike the pull-up, which is typically easier with an underhand grip, performing a muscle-up with your palms facing towards you is much harder than with your palms facing away. In order to perform a reverse grip muscle-up, you need to generate a lot of explosive power by kipping from your hips and creating a large arc with your body as it moves over the bar. Since you can't use a false grip when your palms are facing you, allow your palms to spin around the bar on the way up. Be careful with this move, as it can place a lot of strain on your thumbs during the transition. At first, you may need to rest your chest on the bar in order to bring your hands around.

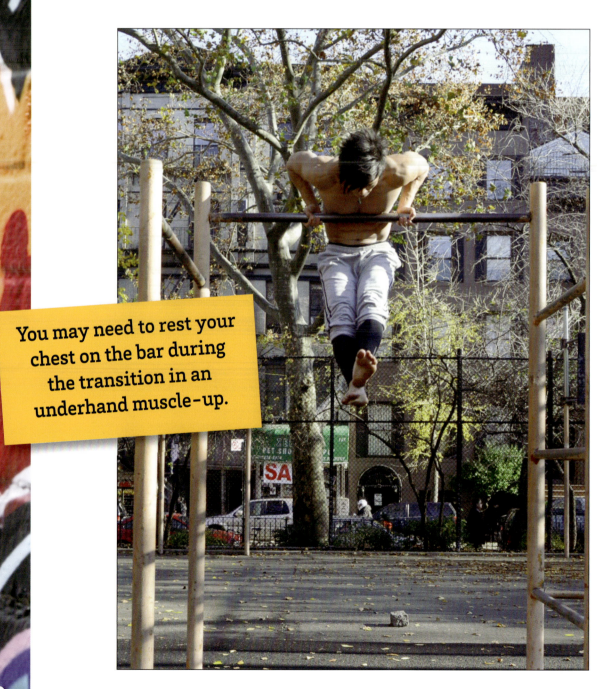

You may need to rest your chest on the bar during the transition in an underhand muscle-up.

X Muscle-up

As the name implies, this variation involves crossing your arms like an X, with each hand over the opposite side's shoulder. When you do an X muscle-up, the arm that is on the bottom has to do most of the work, so start by learning with your dominant side underneath. It took me lots of practice to get the hang of these and I still need to work on cleaning up my form. Even if you are very good at muscle-ups, you're unlikely to get this one on your first try.

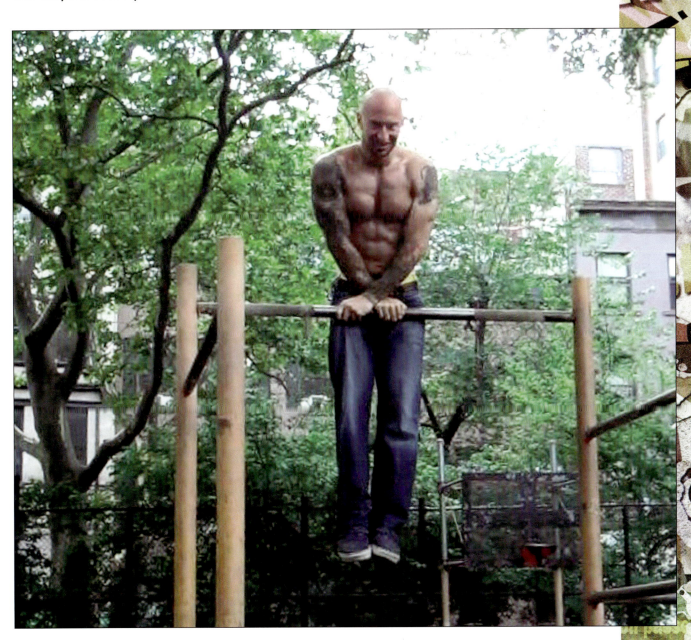

Switchblade Muscle-up

The switch grip or "switchblade" muscle-up is one of the more difficult plyometric variations. To perform the switchblade, start out hanging below the bar in an underhand (chin-up) grip. From here, pull yourself up explosively, reversing your grip during the transition phase. You'll have to generate lots of explosive force to get high enough over the bar to catch yourself and push through the dip phase to complete the exercise.

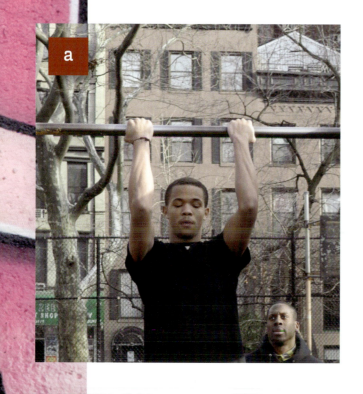
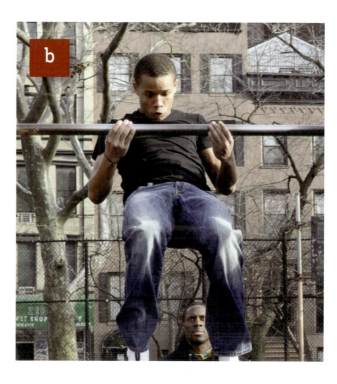
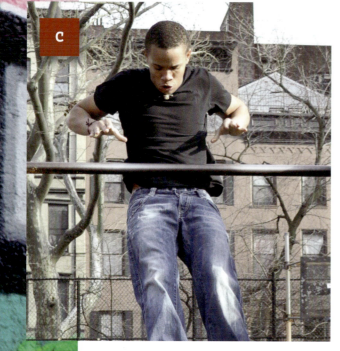
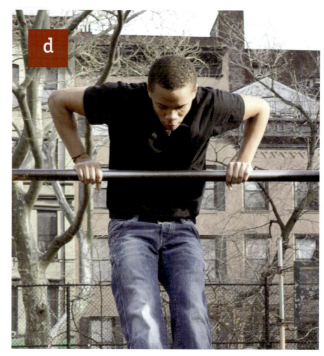

Raising the Bar

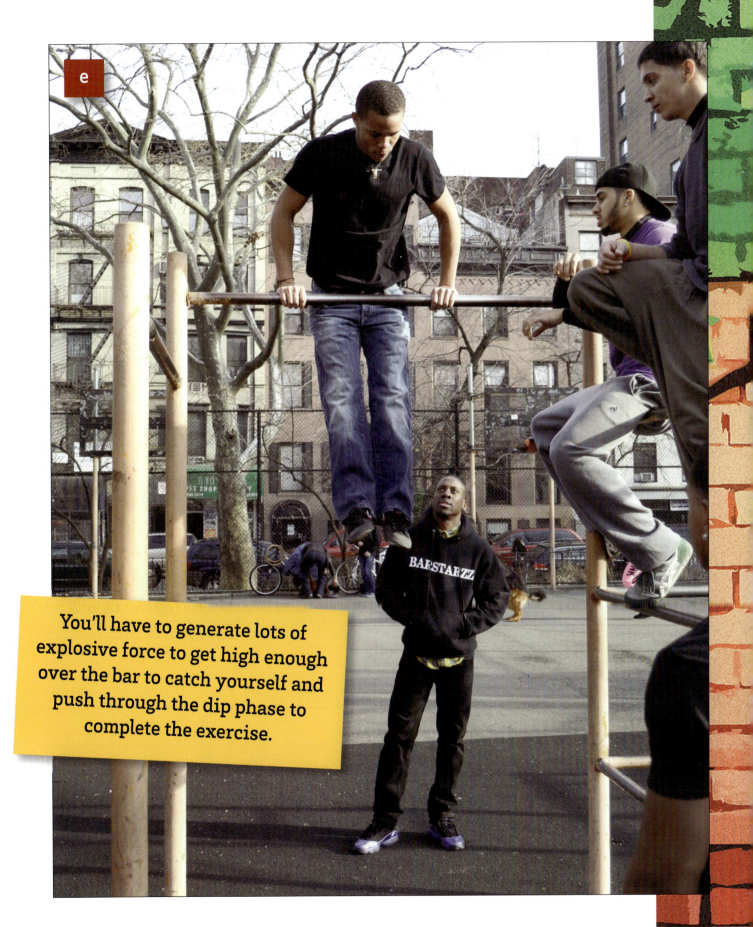

You'll have to generate lots of explosive force to get high enough over the bar to catch yourself and push through the dip phase to complete the exercise.

360 Muscle-up

This move involves releasing the bar at the top of the muscle-up and rotating your entire body in a full 360 degree spin before grabbing the bar on the way down. Moves like the 360 muscle-up look really bad-ass but like a lot of the freestyle variations, they aren't necessary for someone who's simply looking to get strong and fit. With increased difficulty sometimes comes increased risk. (I'll come back to this idea later.)

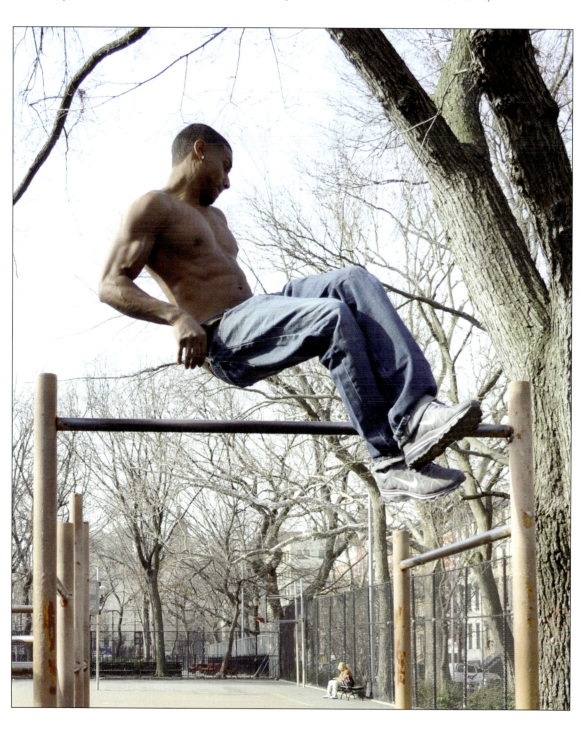

One Arm Muscle-up

While most people (myself included) may never even be close to performing a one arm muscle-up, it is within the spectrum of human possibility. One need look no further than a simple YouTube search for evidence of this. While a few chosen ones might be able to eventually conquer this move, for the rest of us, it should serve to keep us humble and motivated. I mean, if there's someone out there who can do a muscle-up with just one arm, shouldn't any able bodied two armed-man be able to get at least a couple of reps with both?

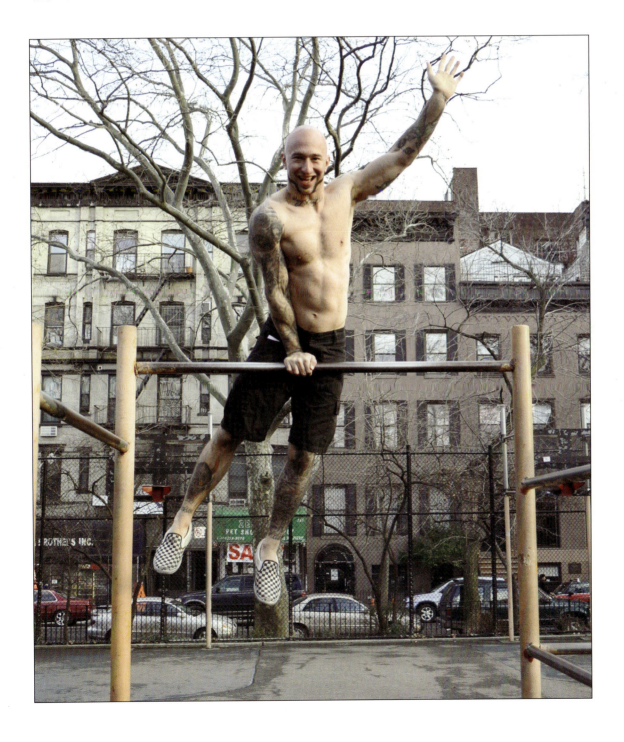

Raising the Bar

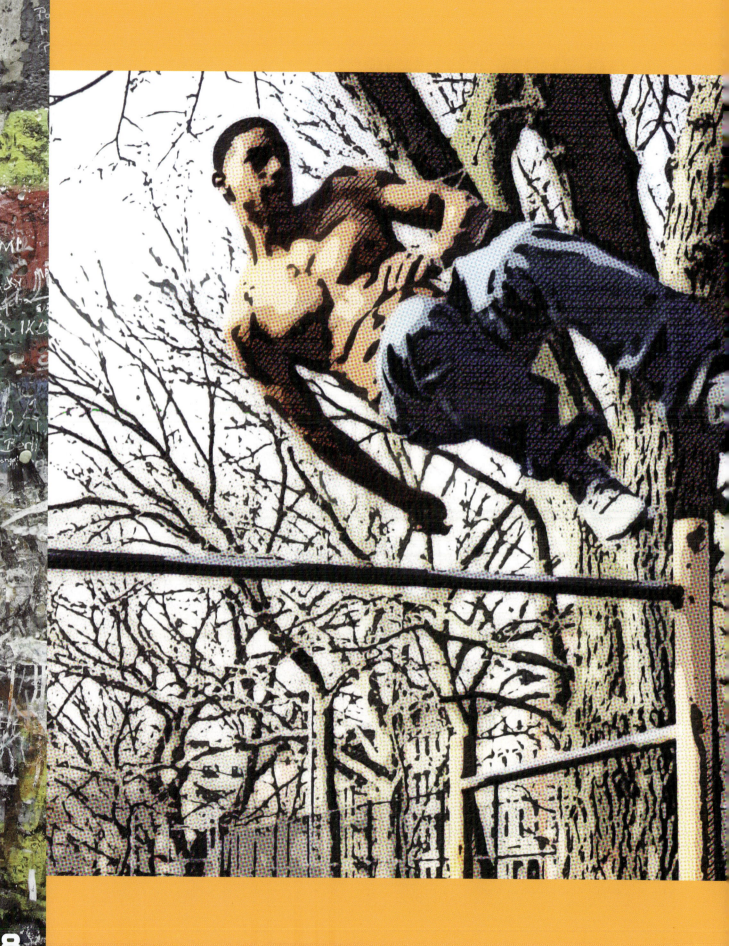

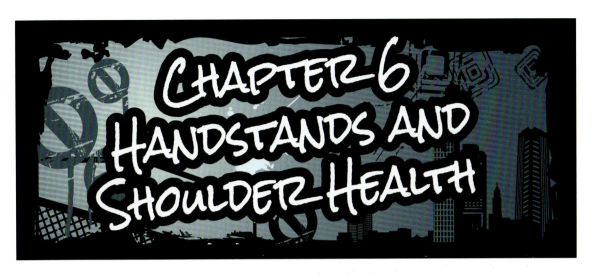

Chapter 6
Handstands and Shoulder Health

"To every action there is always an equal and opposite reaction."
–Sir Isaac Newton

The world can be a confusing and complicated place, but one thing remains true. The universe will always strive to maintain balance in order to sustain itself. Your body is no different, it too must maintain balance between opposing muscle groups in order to function properly. Practicing handstands can help you achieve that balance (pun intended).

Seriously though, if you do pull-ups all the time and don't work any overhead pressing into your routine you will undoubtedly be setting yourself up for shoulder problems, including limited range of motion, poor posture, impinged tendons or worse.

Yep, you've gotta do some kind of overhead pressing to keep you're joints healthy. The most common way to do this is with weights, in which case you'll have to join a gym or get a set of dumbbells, barbells or kettlebells to keep in your home. The alternative, of course, is to practice handstands. Not only can handstands build strength and endurance in your shoulders, they also provide an active stretch for the lats. Hand-balancing also improves neurological function and body awareness. Additionally, inverted positions are excellent for the body's circulation.

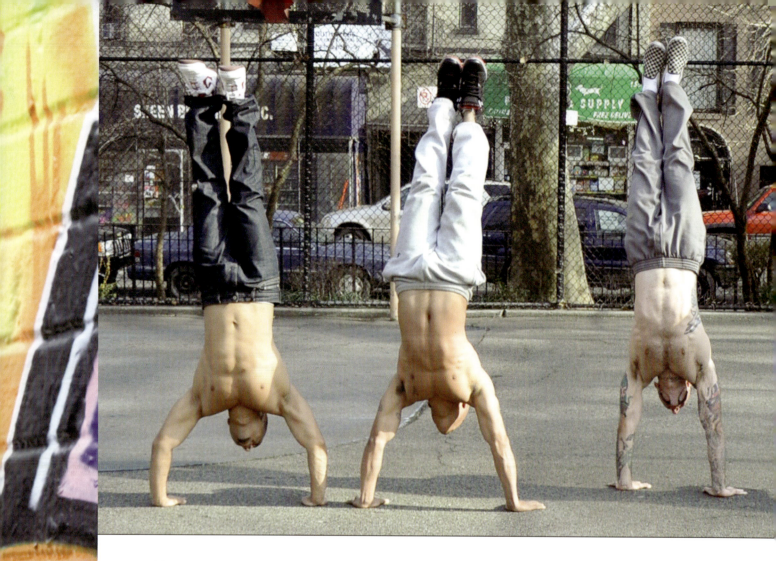

Shoulder Rollouts

Before you begin handstand practice, I recommend that you prep your shoulders by performing shoulder rollouts. Though this exercise is often referred to as a shoulder dislocation, practicing these should actually make your shoulder joints stronger and less likely to dislocate, so I call them shoulder rollouts.

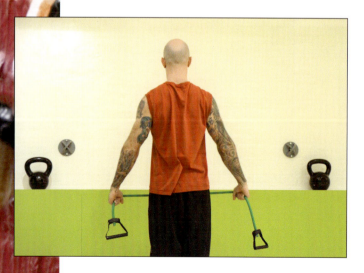

It is also worth noting that this is the only exercise discussed in this book in which I recommend a piece of equipment other than a bar. A rubber stretch band is the best thing to use for these.

Hold the stretch band in front of you with your hands just wider than hip distance. Pull your hands outward to create some tension on the band. From here reach your arms up overhead and bring them all the way around to the other side.

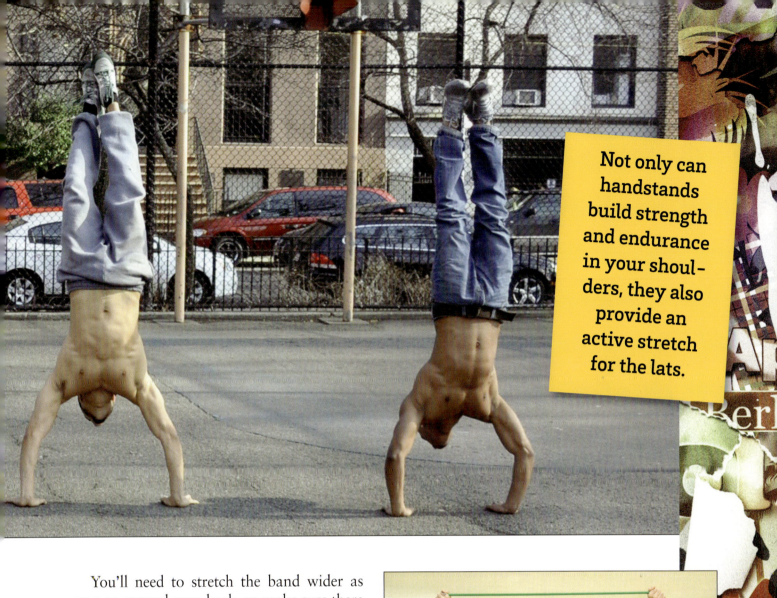

Not only can handstands build strength and endurance in your shoulders, they also provide an active stretch for the lats.

You'll need to stretch the band wider as you go around your back, so make sure there is enough slack on your band to allow you to do this. Just like when you're doing pull-ups, be careful not to let your shoulders shrug upward as your arms go overhead.

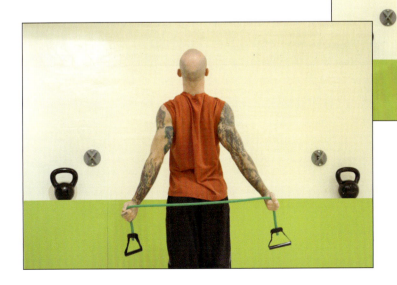

Don't let your shoulders shrug upward as your arms go overhead.

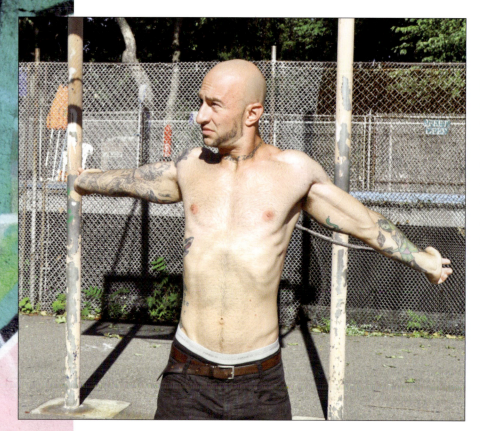

Shoulder rollouts are actually a great warm-up before any upperbody workout. I highly recommend that you make them a regular part of your fitness regimen. If you don't have access to a rubber exercise band, you can use a stick or other long, lightweight object. Backward arm circles are another good substitute for those of you looking to avoid additional equipment.

Kick-up

In the beginning, you've got a few things that you can practice concurrently in order to build to a freestanding handstand. The first thing to try is kicking up into a handstand against a wall.

Start out by facing the wall, then reach both your hands up over your head and take a small step forward. From here, plant your hands firmly on the ground a few inches away from the wall with your elbows locked as you kick one leg up and then the other. If you can get into the handstand position, try to hold it for several seconds before coming down. Don't push your luck right away though, gradually build up to longer holds. In time, you should aim to hold your handstand as long as possible without coming down. I recommend a minimum of one minute against the wall before you begin working on a freestanding handstand.

If you aren't strong enough (or confident enough) to jump right in with the kick-up method, check out these other suggestions and come back to the kick-up when you feel ready.

RAISING THE BAR

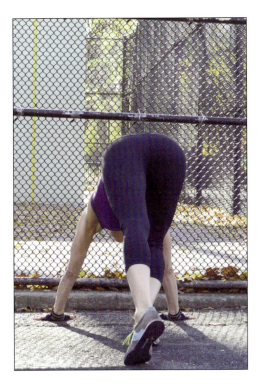
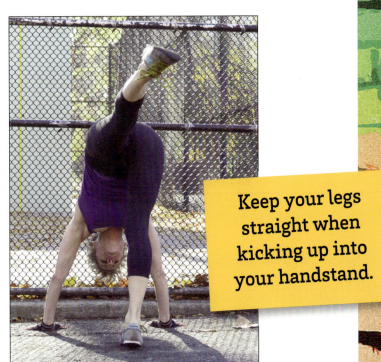

Keep your legs straight when kicking up into your handstand.

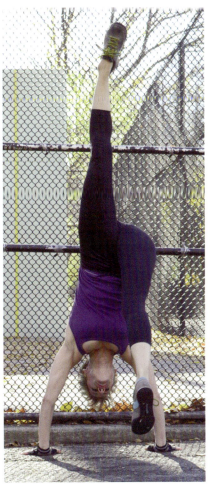
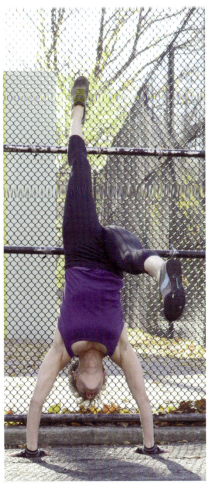
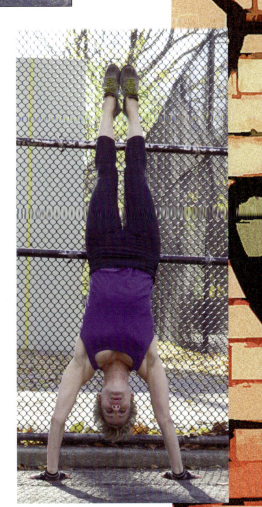

Frogstand

Known as a crow pose in yoga, the frogstand will give you a feel for balancing on your hands, without the instability of having to support your body in a vertical position. To perform a frogstand, squat down and place your hands on the floor with your elbows slightly bent. Next, bring your knees up towards your armpits and rest your shins on the backs of your arms (your triceps). Try to look out rather than down as you tip your weight forward and come off your feet. In the beginning, you can bend your elbows as much as you need to. Think about making a little shelf with your arms for your legs to rest on. In time, you'll be able to straighten out your arms when performing your frogstand. Once you can accomplish this, you'll soon be ready for a freestanding handstand.

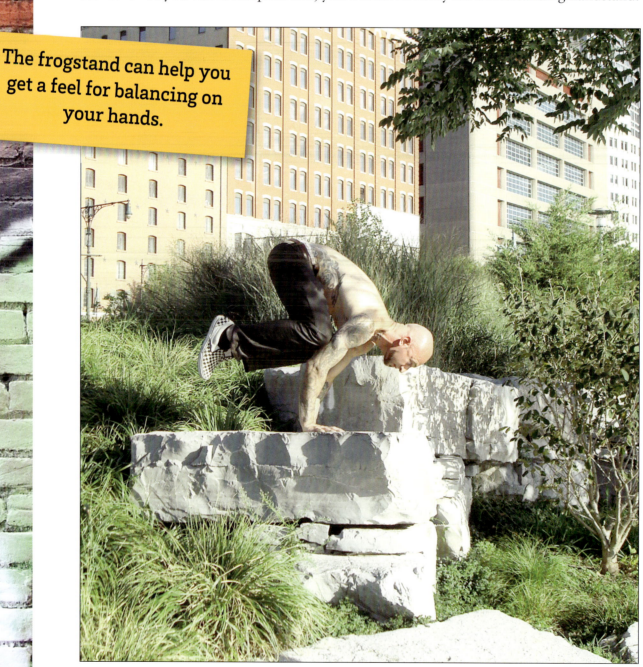

The frogstand can help you get a feel for balancing on your hands.

Wall Walking

Get into a push-up position with your feet at the base of a wall. Now slowly start to walk your feet up the wall as you gradually bring your hands closer towards it. Start by trying to get your hips over your shoulders like an upside-down L-hold. In time you will be able to get your body fully vertical from this position by walking your feet higher up on the wall and bringing your hands closer to it. Once you can do this, kicking up into a handstand should be no problem.

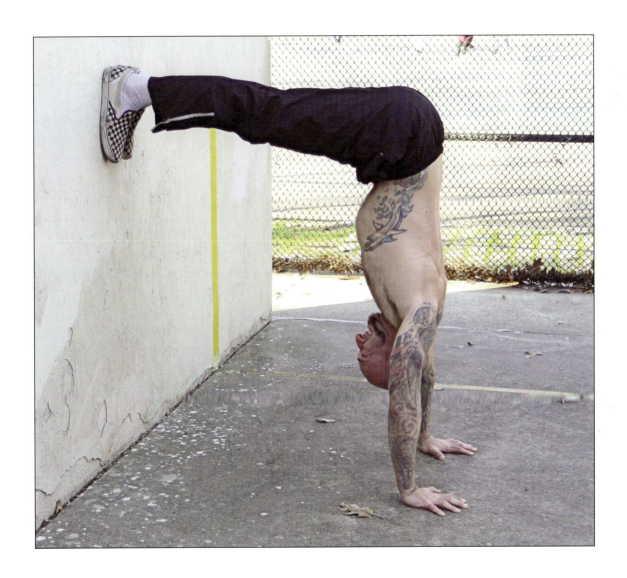

Off The Wall

After several weeks or months of practicing those basics, you should eventually be ready to move up to attempting a freestanding handstand. This can be intimidating because there is nothing to catch you if you fall. You must take a leap of faith and go in with confidence that your body will know what to do if you tip over. If you're having a hard time getting over your nerves, it can help to have a spotter. It's can also be helpful to practice on a soft surface like grass or rubber.

While a free-standing handstand can be a challenging shoulder and arm workout when held for long enough, the balance is typically the most difficult part to learn. It takes a lot of time to find the "sweet spot" between over-balancing (tipping over) or under-balancing (falling back to your feet).

Unlike your foot, which was made for standing, your hand doesn't have a true heel, so it's best to put slightly more weight in your fingers than in your palms when balancing on them. If you are a tiny bit over-balanced, you can stay up by pressing your fingers into the ground. When you're under-balanced, there is less you can do to keep from coming down.

> If you're having a hard time getting over your nerves, it can help to have a spotter.

Raising the Bar

Coming Down

Since the fear of falling can make training the freestanding handstand intimidating, it's important to learn how to come down safely when you lose your balance. The two easiest ways to do this are to kick down, like you would coming down from a wall, or to perform a pirouette, which isn't quite as fancy as it sounds.

If you are in a handstand and you feel yourself losing your balance towards the front of your body (underbalancing), falling to your feet should happen fairly naturally. Just remember to float down gently and maintain straight legs on your descent.

If you feel yourself losing your balance towards the back of your body (overbalancing), the smartest thing to do is lift one hand from the ground and take a small step forward with it. Quickly turn your hips and your body should float down towards your toes. This should also happen somewhat naturally.

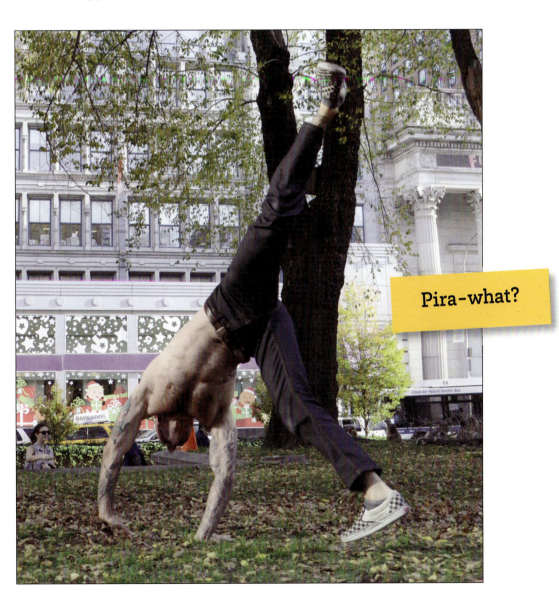

Pira-what?

A Tale of Two Handstands

In modern gymnastics, handstands are performed with a perfectly straight line from top to bottom. For this reason, a lot of people will tell you that arching your back during a handstand is bad form. In my experience, however, it is helpful to allow your back to arch while you are learning to find the balance. In time, you can work on reaching your legs upward, pressing into the floor and tightening your abs, lower back and glutes to achieve an aesthetically pleasing straight line from head to toe (or hands to toe as the case may be). Though in theory, a perfectly straight handstand can require less effort to hold in terms of muscular output, the balance is harder to find, especially for people who have limited shoulder mobility. Aim towards the eventual goal of a totally straight handstand, but til then, just try to find the balance wherever you can.

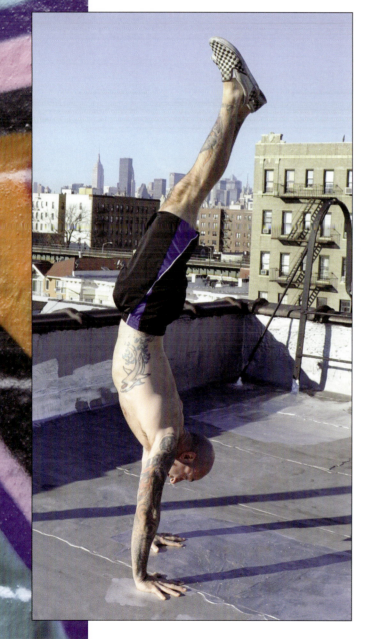
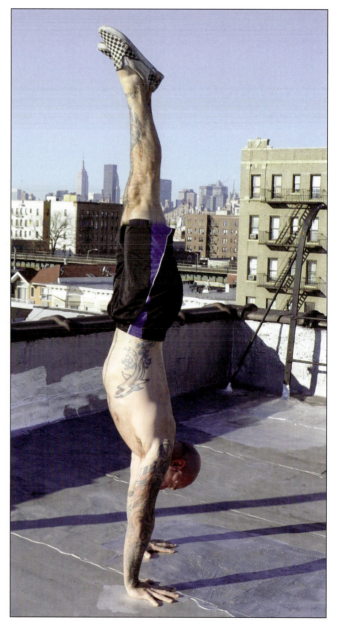

Keep Practicing

Transitioning from a handstand against a wall to a free standing handstand is a challenging and potentially discouraging process. I was terrible at hand balancing when I started out, but I've been practicing for a while now. For me, the key has been consistency; I rarely miss a day of practice, even if it's just a couple of minutes at the end of a workout. Some days it comes harder than others, but when I fall, I just get up and try again.

Press To Handstand

The press to handstand is a much more challenging way to get into a freestanding handstand. There are a few different ways to approach it.

The simplest variation is to begin in a frogstand and try to press yourself by extending your legs as you press with your shoulders and arms.

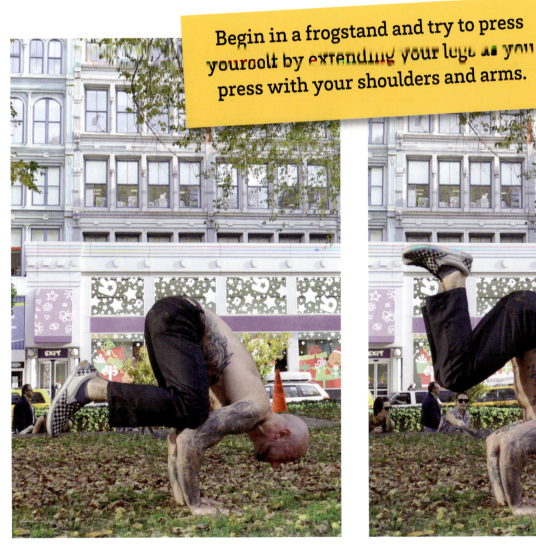
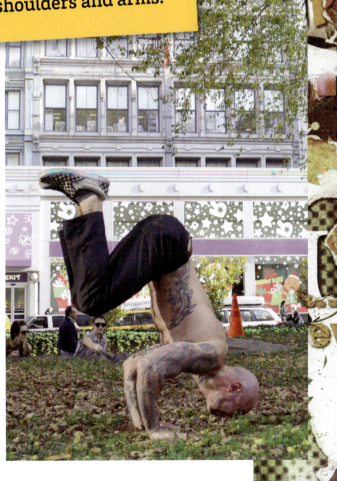

> Begin in a frogstand and try to press yourself by extending your legs as you press with your shoulders and arms.

RAISING THE BAR

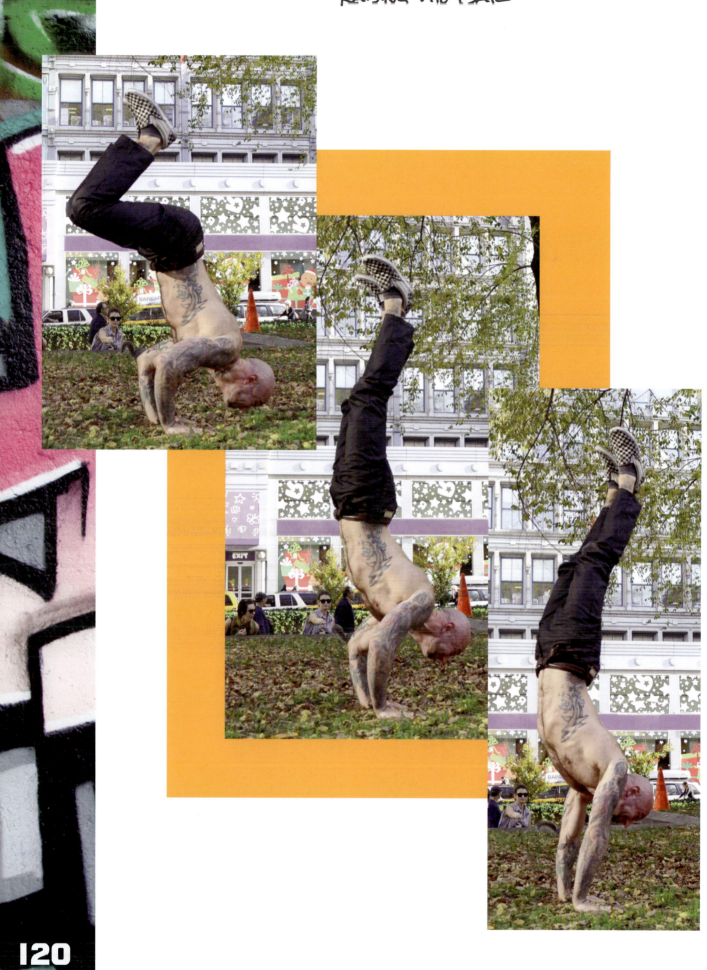

120

Raising the Bar

You can also press to a handstand from your feet, by bending over, placing your hands on the ground, and shifting your weight forward into your palms. Engage your core as you raise your legs up. This takes lots of practice and requires better than average flexibility, so keep at it! This can be done from a normal standing position or with your legs in a straddle.

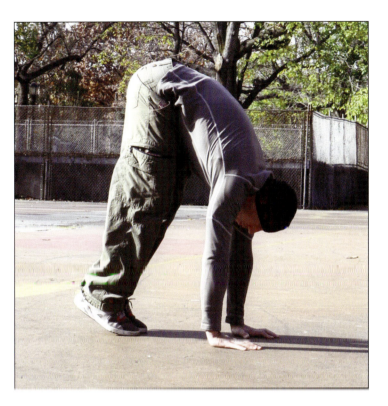

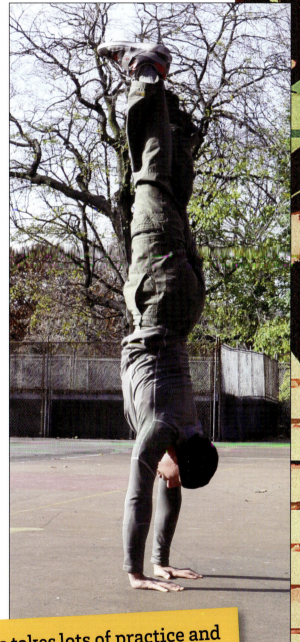

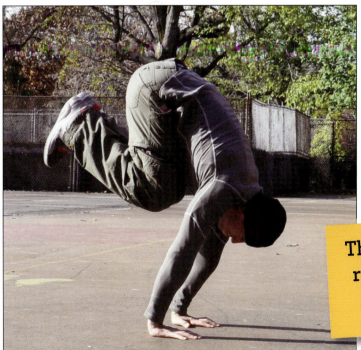

This takes lots of practice and requires better than average flexibility, so keep at it!

Raising the Bar

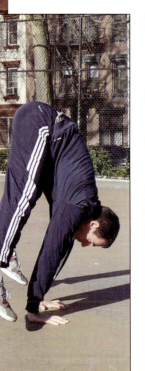
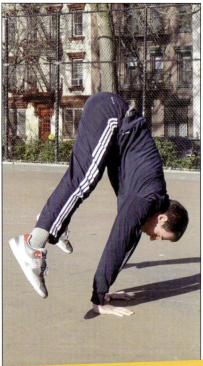
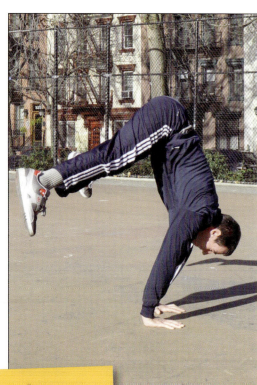

Engage your core as you raise your legs up.

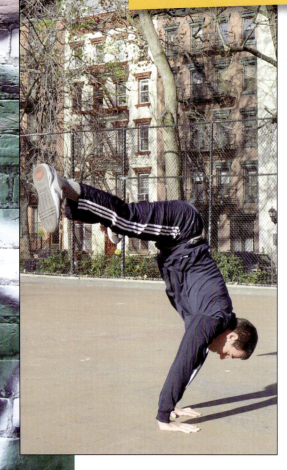
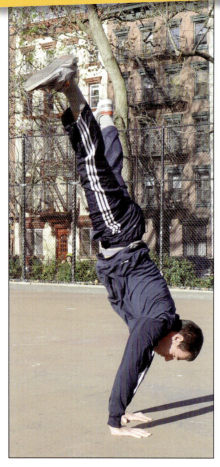
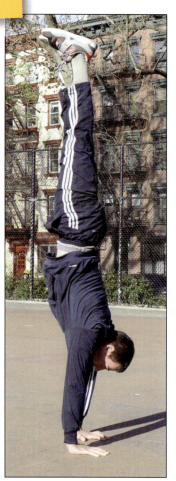

Handstands on the Bars

Though I recommend learning to do a handstand on the ground first, handstands can be performed on bars or other objects once you reach a certain level of comfort. Performing a handstand on a straight bar or parallel bars requires tremendous control as well as grip strength. Straight bars and parallel bars are both good choices for practicing this move, though each is challenging in unique ways. Either way, get a feel for the handstand on a low bar(s) first before trying it up high. You'll need to learn to safely bail out of this move and land on your feet without hurting yourself before going for it on the high bar.

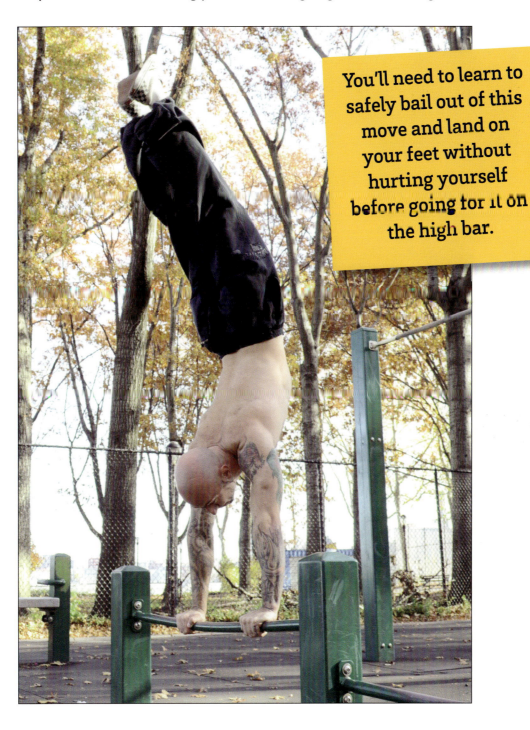

You'll need to learn to safely bail out of this move and land on your feet without hurting yourself before going for it on the high bar.

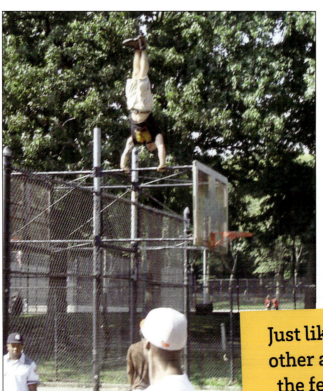

If you're going to do a handstand on a high bar, you'll have to get up there first by performing a muscle-up or a rollover. From there, it's a lot like the press to handstand discussed earlier. Just like muscle-overs and other advanced bar moves, the fear factor is high for moves like this one. And for good reason - try this stuff at your own risk!

> Just like muscle-overs and other advanced bar moves, the fear factor is high for moves like this one.

One Handed Handstand

The ultimate handbalancing progression is the one handed handstand. To even hold this move for one entire second can take lots of practice. Only once you can hold a normal freestanding handstand for a full minute should you begin training the one handed version.

When going for a one handed handstand, begin by getting into a standard two hand handstand first. From here slowly shift your weight towards one side as you spread your legs for balance. (Hip mobility play a big part in this, so make sure to practice your straddle on the ground as well.) Start by trying to touch your hand to your shoulder quickly before returning it to the ground. Eventually you might be able to stay on one hand a bit longer. You may find it helpful to reach your free arm away from your body for balance. Advanced handbalancers can get their entire body straight over just one hand.

Raising the Bar

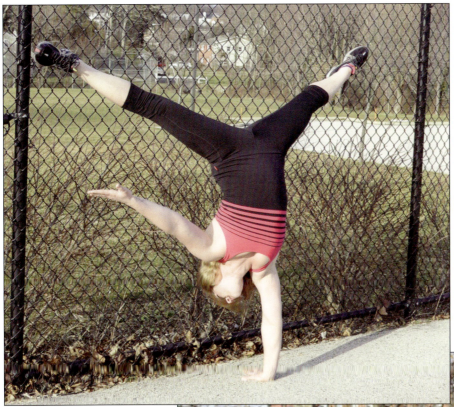

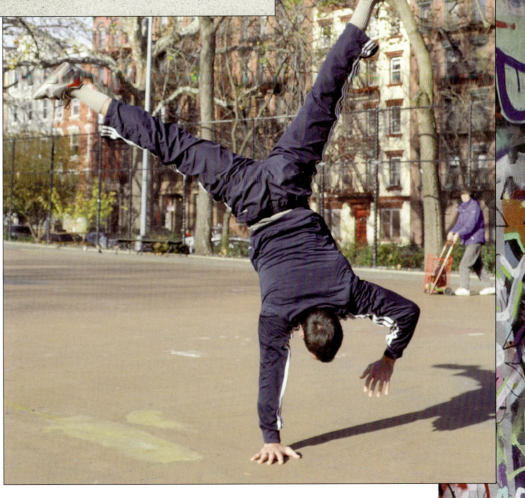

Raising the Bar

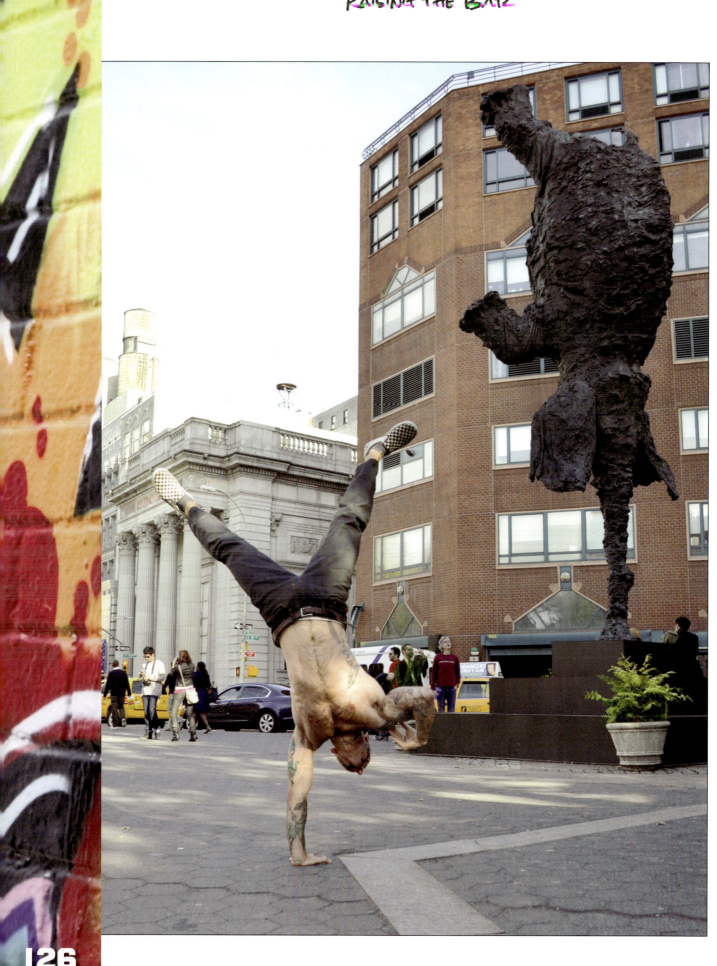

Raising the Bar

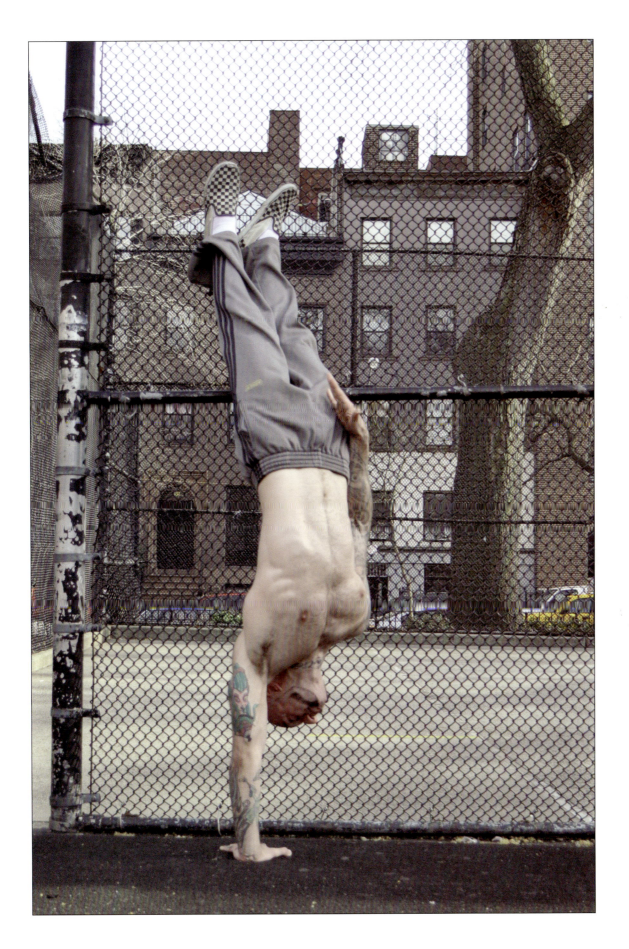

Handstand Push-ups

In addition to just holding handstands, doing handstand push-ups (and handstand push-up variations) is also essential. After all, you need to work those muscles through a full range of motion!

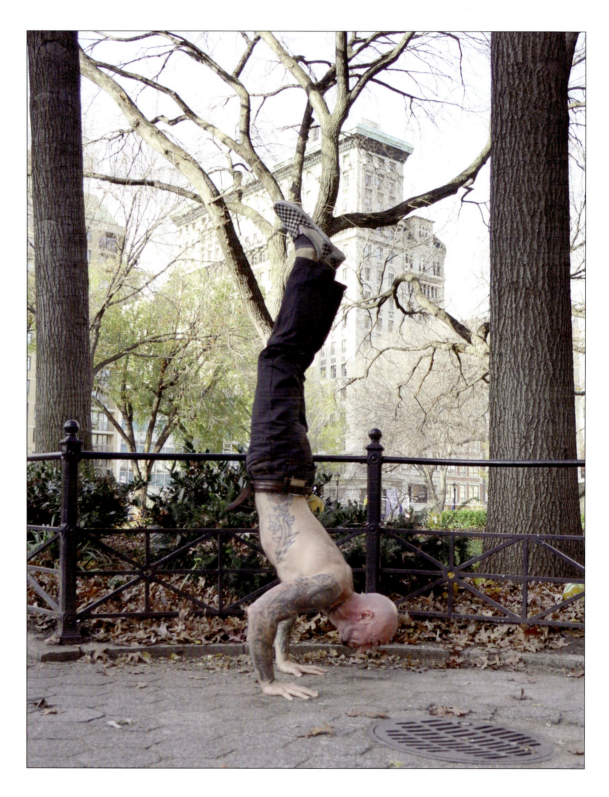

Pike Push-up

If you aren't strong enough to do a full handstand push-up yet, the pike push-up is a great way to ease in. Pike push-ups allow you to train the movement pattern without having to bear your entire body weight.

Rest your toes on a bench or step and get down in a push-up position. From here, walk your hands back toward the bench while you pike your hips up in the air over your shoulders. (The position is very similar to the upside-down L shape we discussed a few pages back.) Make sure to keep your back straight by taking the stretch in your hamstrings, though you may bend your knees a little if you need to in order to keep your hips up over your shoulders. Lower yourself down until the top of your head touches the ground and then push yourself back up – that's one rep.

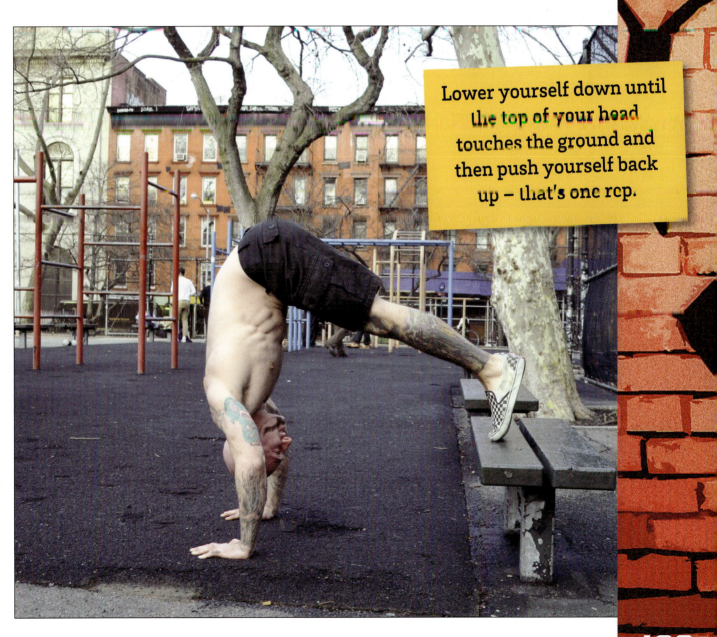

Lower yourself down until the top of your head touches the ground and then push yourself back up – that's one rep.

Wall Assisted Handstand Push-up

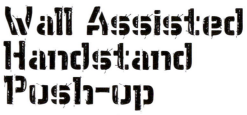

Once you can do ten consecutive pike presses without too much trouble, you're ready to try a full handstand push-up against a wall. Kick up into a handstand with your back slightly arched. Engage your core muscles and keep your body tight as you lower yourself down and press yourself back up. Make sure you touch your head to the ground on every rep to ensure a full range of motion. You can also try touching your nose to the floor instead of the top of your head to allow yourself to go a bit lower.

> Once you can do ten consecutive pike presses without too much trouble, you're ready to try a full handstand pushup against a wall.

Freestanding Handstand Push-up

The freestanding handstand is a tricky move to get the hang of on its own, adding a push-up to it takes things to a whole other level!

The freestanding handstand push-up requires tremendous strength, balance and total body control, so before you think about training for this move, I suggest getting to the point where you can do at least ten wall assisted handstand push-ups and hold a freestanding handstand for a full minute.

When performing handstand holds, I've often found it helpful to look in between my hands. With the freestanding handstand push-up however, I've found it better to look a few inches in front of my hands. Since the balance changes throughout the range of motion, I recommend practicing static holds at the bottom and middle positions to help train for this feat. When a freestanding handstand push-up is performed on the bar, it is quite a sight to behold!

Raising the Bar

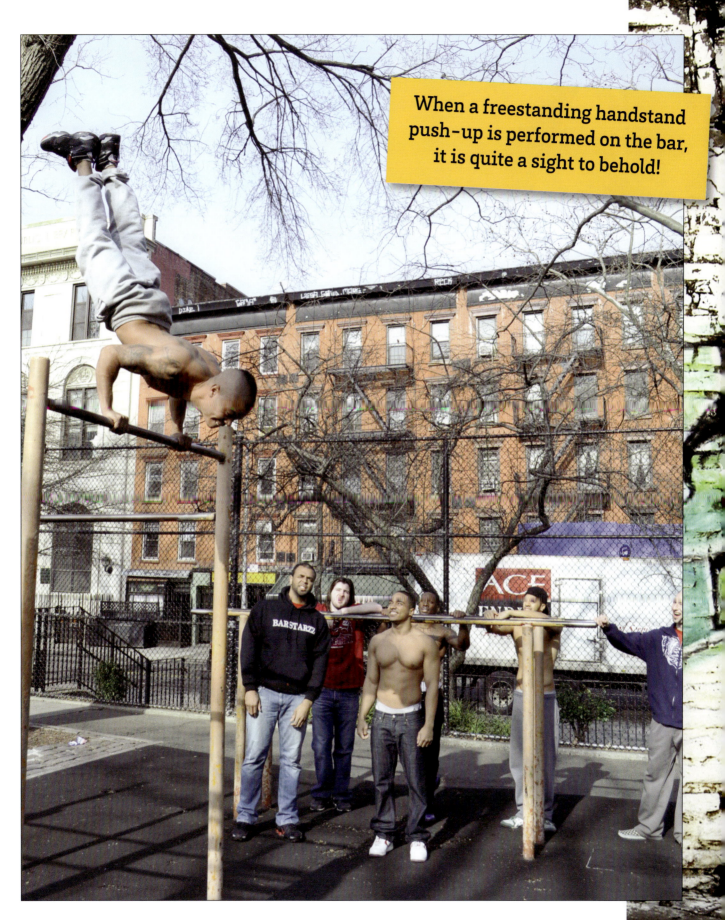

When a freestanding handstand push-up is performed on the bar, it is quite a sight to behold!

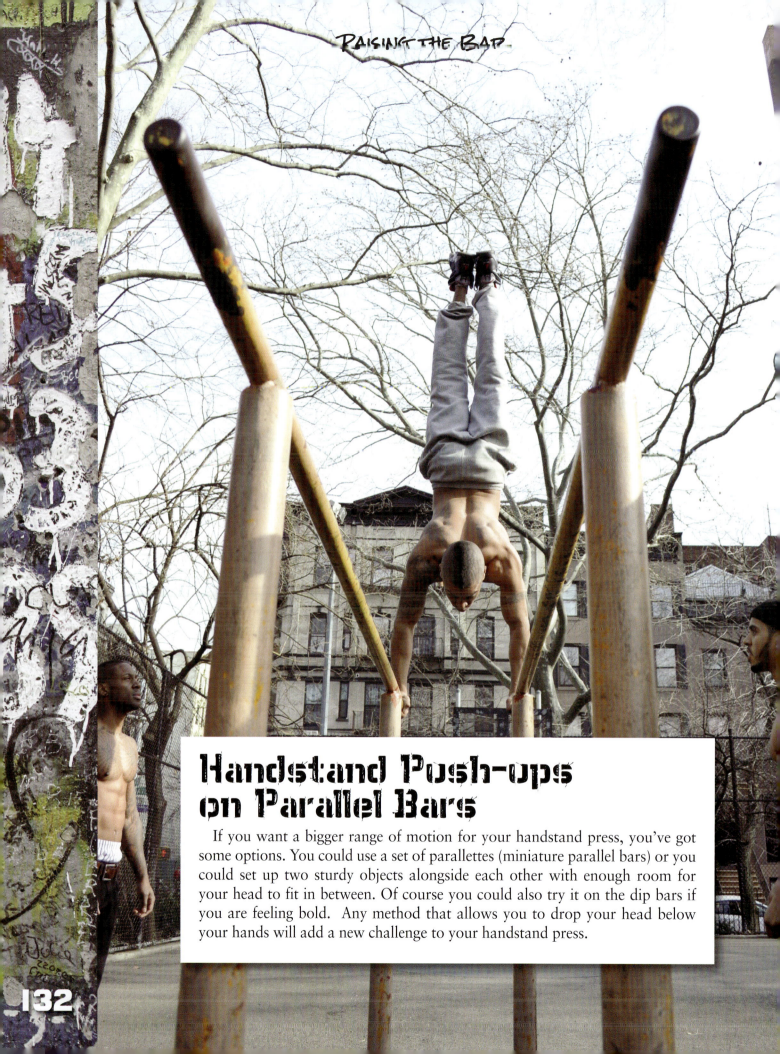

Handstand Push-ups on Parallel Bars

If you want a bigger range of motion for your handstand press, you've got some options. You could use a set of parallettes (miniature parallel bars) or you could set up two sturdy objects alongside each other with enough room for your head to fit in between. Of course you could also try it on the dip bars if you are feeling bold. Any method that allows you to drop your head below your hands will add a new challenge to your handstand press.

Raising the Bar

The One Arm Handstand Push-up

Often discussed, though never actually executed, the one arm handstand push-up is the holy grail of bodyweight strength training.

In theory, the one arm handstand push-up is the ultimate calisthenics exercise. However, a full, clean rep has never been documented as far as I know. I have no doubt that someone will eventually perform one (and get it on video), but in the meantime the rest of us will just have to continue to train hard and keep the dream alive.

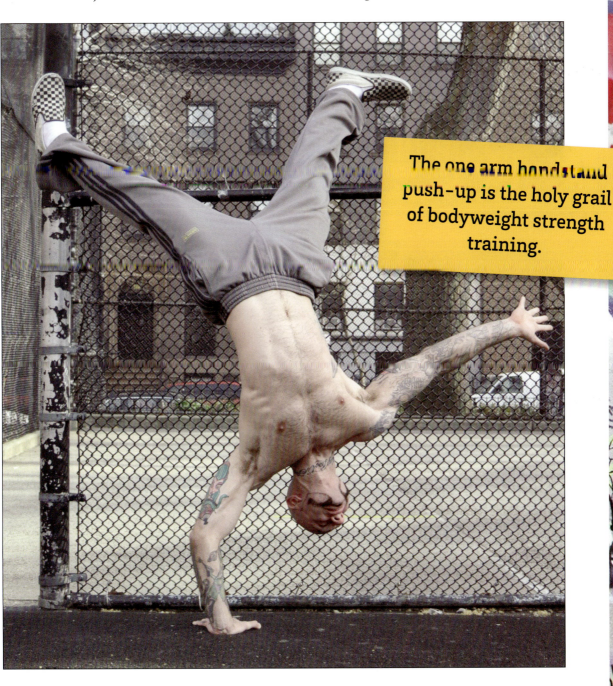

The one arm handstand push-up is the holy grail of bodyweight strength training.

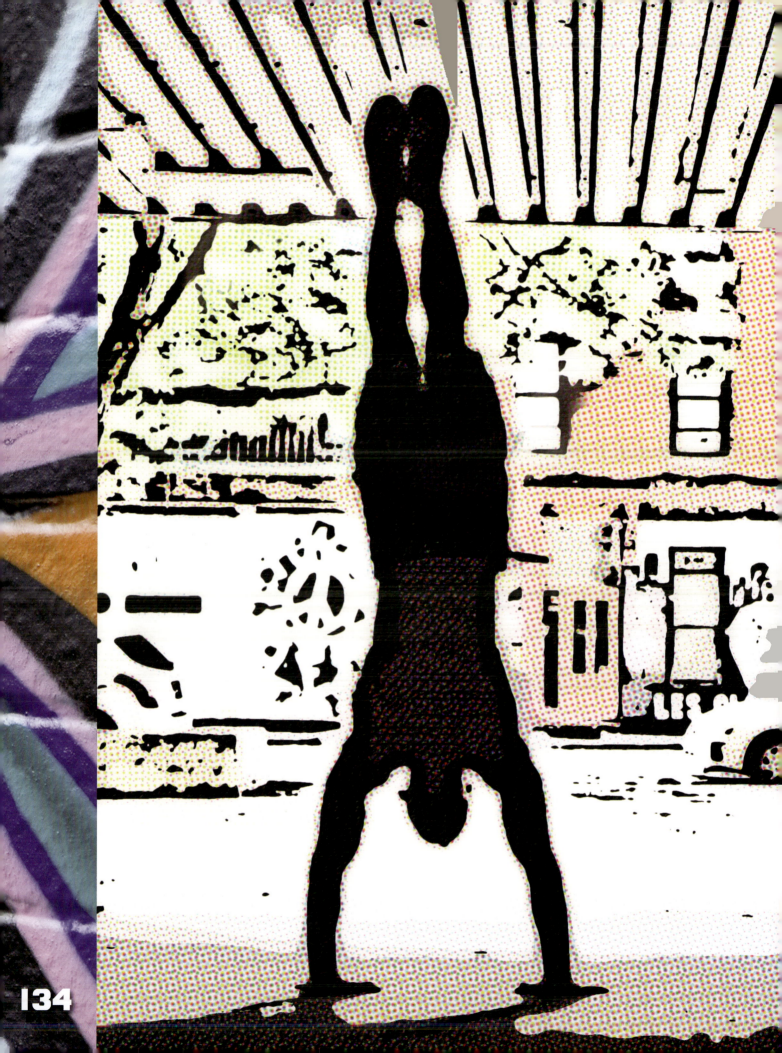

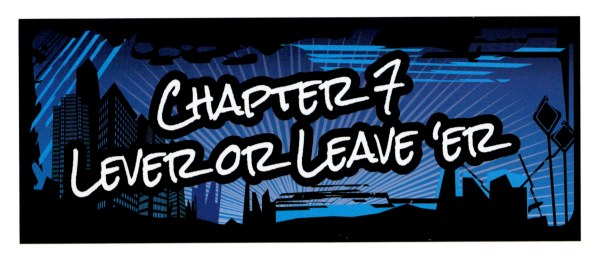

CHAPTER 7
LEVER OR LEAVE 'ER

> "Don't ask what the world needs.
> Ask what makes you come alive,
> and go do it. Because what the world
> needs is people who have come alive."
> –Howard Thurman

Performing a body lever is no easy task. Even once you're already proficient in pull-ups and muscle-ups, it can still take months or years to achieve a solid lever hold. You better really love bodyweight training if you are going to embark down this road. Only those of you who have a burning passion for building bodyweight strength should proceed.

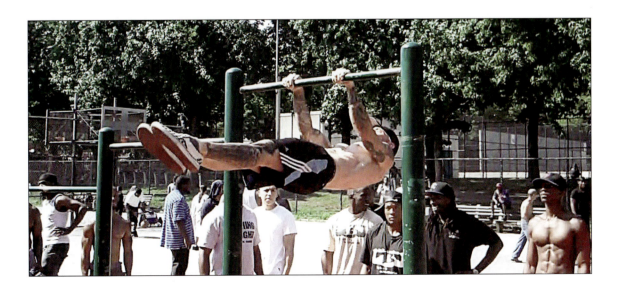

Levers (especially the front lever) are among the most challenging bodyweight exercises out there. They require tremendous core strength as well as a powerful upper-body. Practicing towards these movements can build serious strength in your arms, chest, back and abs. Levers also train you to use your muscles to work together, which is how to utilize them most effectively. Let's check out the different types of levers that you can perform on the bar.

Elbow Lever

This is one of the only non-bar exercises I've included in this book, though like the handstand, it can be performed on a bar when a high level of confidence and comfort have been attained. As the name implies, an elbow lever is performed by leveraging your bodyweight against one or both elbows while balancing on your hand(s) with your body stretched out in a horizontal position. Though it looks similar to a gymnastics planche, the elbow lever is a less difficult skill due to the fact that your upper-body is resting on your arm(s).

While an elbow lever can be performed on a variety of surfaces, I recommend starting out by practicing on a bench, step or any other flat, raised object. This will allow you to wrap your fingers around the side of the object, which most people will find a bit easier than using a flat handed grip.

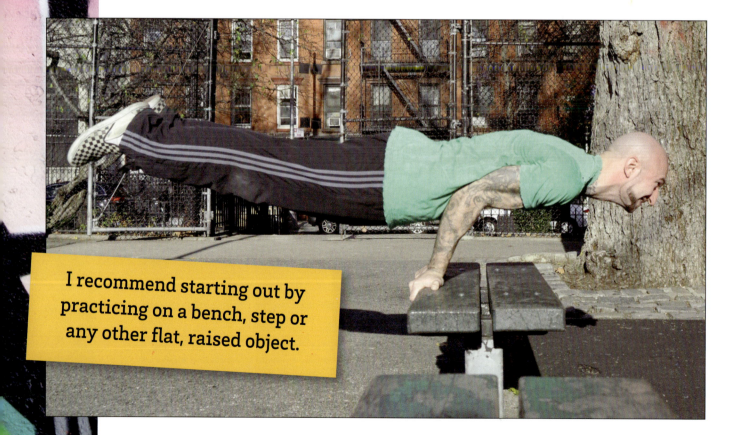

I recommend starting out by practicing on a bench, step or any other flat, raised object.

The other advantage of practicing on a bench is that it allows for more room to lift your legs into position, as opposed to the limited amount of space when starting with your hands on the floor. This will give you more wiggle room to play with the balance.

Make sure to keep your abs contracted and engage your lower back as you raise yourself into position. It is also important to pitch your upper-body forward in order to counterbalance the weight of your bottom half. Your elbows will likely need to be extended beyond ninety degrees in order to achieve a solid elbow lever hold. Note the positioning of my elbows and hands in the photo below:

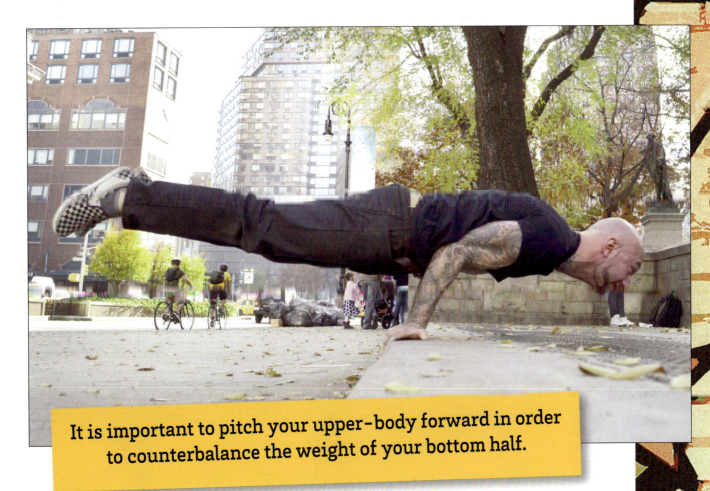

It is important to pitch your upper-body forward in order to counterbalance the weight of your bottom half.

When practicing the elbow lever, you'll want to position your elbows right up against your hip bones. Concentrate on squeezing your midsection tight as you lift up into position, as some of your elbow will inevitably wind up against your stomach. It may take some time to get used to the sensation of having your elbows jutting into your abdomen; beginners tend to find it especially unpleasant. With practice, however, you can eventually learn to make peace with the feeling.

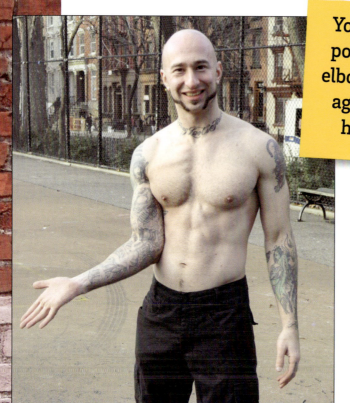 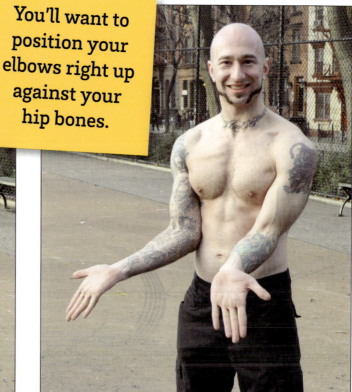

> You'll want to position your elbows right up against your hip bones.

As it is a hand-balancing skill, the elbow lever can also be a useful tool in working towards a freestanding handstand. It's a nice intermediary step between the frogstand and handstand.

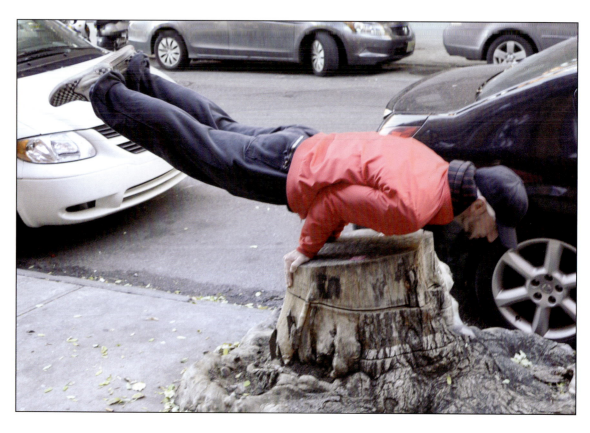

One Arm Elbow Lever

Though break-dancers and other skilled hand-balancers have a way of making this move seem effortless, the one arm elbow lever is a very challenging feat, so be patient if you endeavor to add this one to your arsenal.

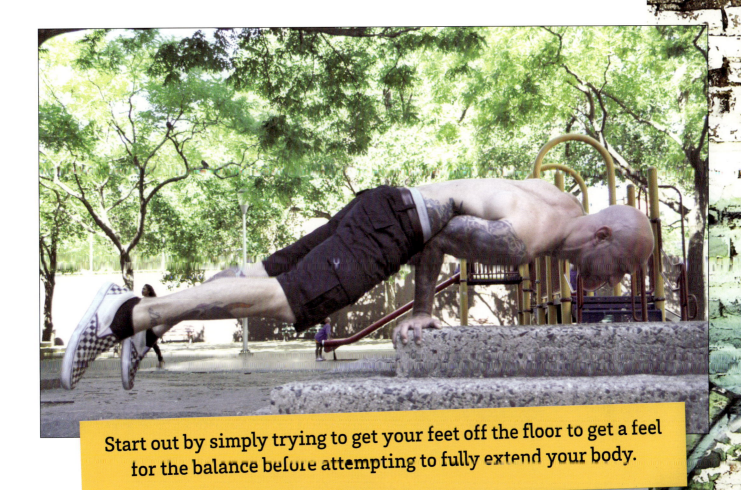

Start out by simply trying to get your feet off the floor to get a feel for the balance before attempting to fully extend your body.

Just like the two arm version, start out by simply trying to get your feet off the floor to get a feel for the balance before attempting to fully extend your body. It is helpful to spot yourself with your free hand in the beginning by reaching it to the side and resting one or several fingers on the surface upon which you are balancing. From here you can try to take the hand away for a second to get a momentary feel for the full exercise, eventually removing it altogether.

There are a couple of subtleties to performing an elbow lever that are unique to the one arm version. First off, it can help to rotate your body away from the ground slightly when performing this variation to prevent yourself from tipping over to that side. You want your weight evenly distributed on both sides of your hand.

Raising the Bar

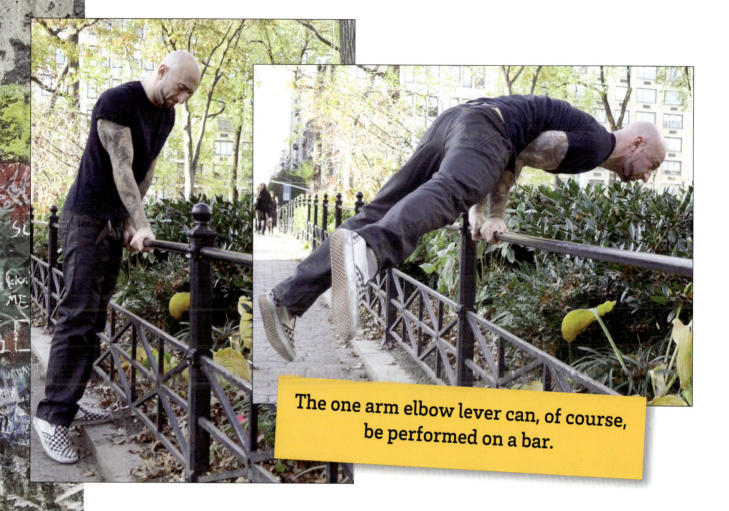

The one arm elbow lever can, of course, be performed on a bar.

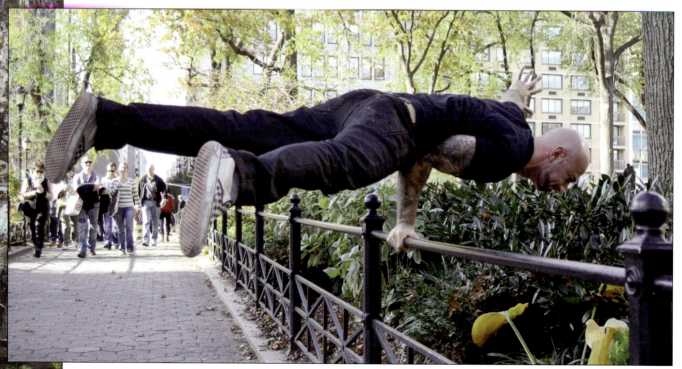

RAISING THE BAR

Additionally, holding your body in a triangular formation with your legs in a straddle can also make it a bit easier to find the balance with this exercise. With practice, you'll improve to the point where you can work on bringing your body into a straight line.

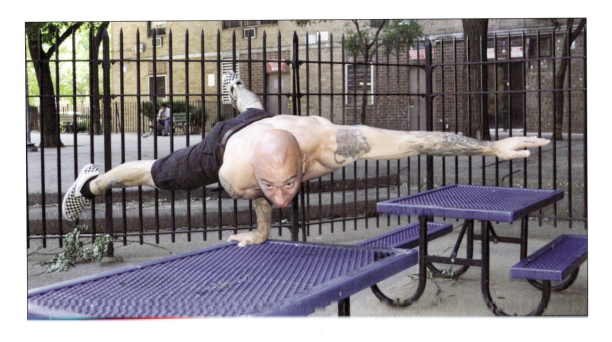

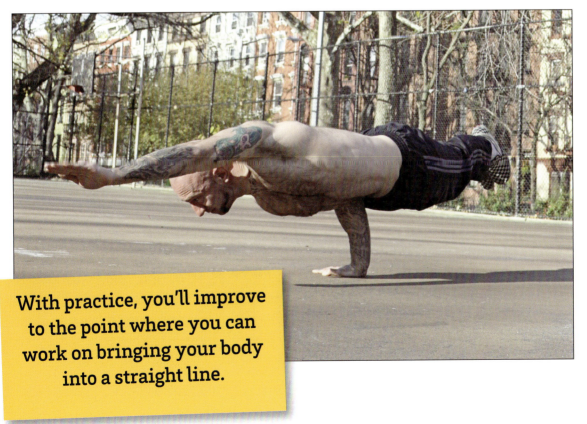

With practice, you'll improve to the point where you can work on bringing your body into a straight line.

Back Levers

Man has yet to fly without airplanes or helicopters, but performing a back lever feels pretty close! Practicing this exercise can help you build total body strength while giving you the sensation of being suspended in mid-air. Back levers are fun and functional, plus they look bad-ass!

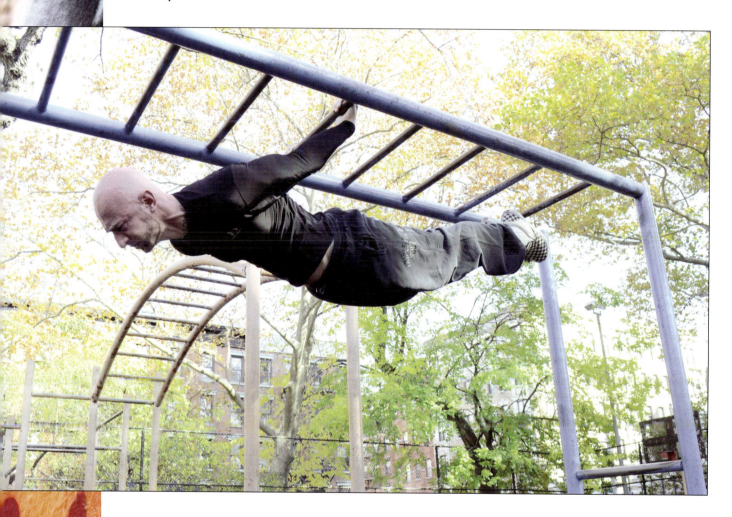

High Angle Back Lever

The way I learned to do a back lever begins by bringing your legs around the bar from a pull-up position, just like skinning the cat. Once your legs are on the other side of the bar, straighten out your entire body so you're hanging almost completely upside down. Your legs will wind up above the bar and your torso will be below.

From here, the objective is to get your body parallel to the ground with your hips directly under the bar, so pitch your chest forward as you lower your legs down. In addition to keeping your abs tight and extending your back, think about actively pulling your hands down towards your hips, engaging your lats, triceps and chest muscles.

Back levers can be performed with a pronated or supinated grip, though I prefer to use an overhand position. It's actually the only way I can do it! Keeping a relatively narrow grip is also a good idea as it allows you to leverage some of your weight against your arms. Think about squeezing your lats and your triceps together to keep yourself up as you suck in your abs, contract your glutes and squeeze your hamstrings.

It's helpful to have someone watch you or videotape you while you are doing this as you'll likely have a hard time feeling when you are in position. (That's actually true for every single exercise in this book.) As always, total body tension is key. Remember to contract your abs, lower back, hamstrings and glutes while performing a back lever. Your arms are only one part of the equation.

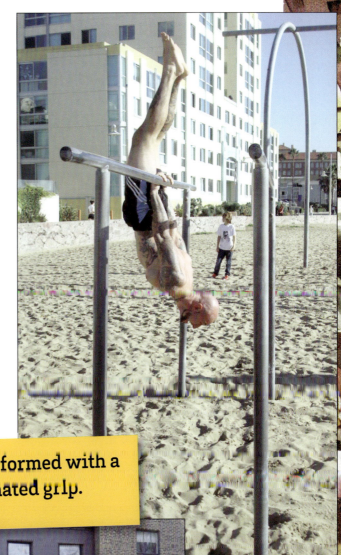

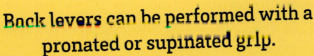

Back levers can be performed with a pronated or supinated grip.

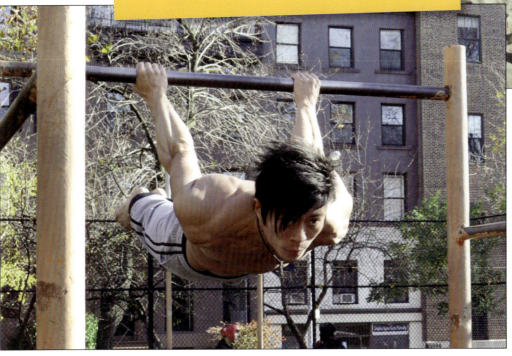

Bent Knee Back Lever

Practicing your back lever with your knees bent will make the move a bit easier, so it's a great way for newcomers to get a feel for the exercise. Other than the knees being bent, everything else is pretty much the same.

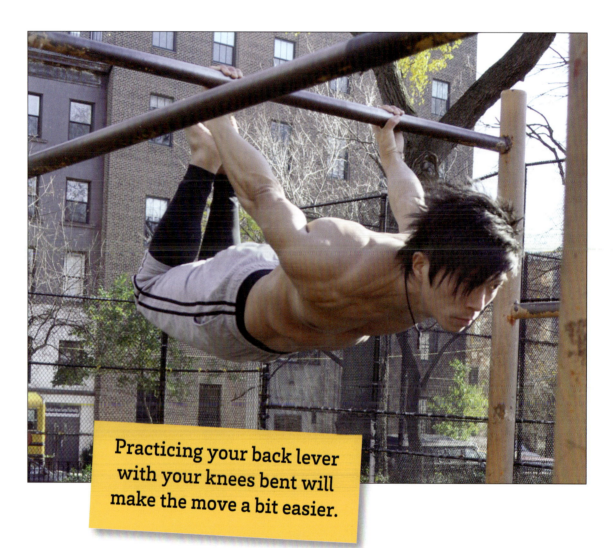

Practicing your back lever with your knees bent will make the move a bit easier.

Front Levers

The front lever is one of the most difficult (and coolest looking) calisthenics exercises out there. Performed either as a static hold or for reps from a hanging position, the front lever involves pulling your whole body up til it's parallel to the floor, almost like you are laying down...on air!

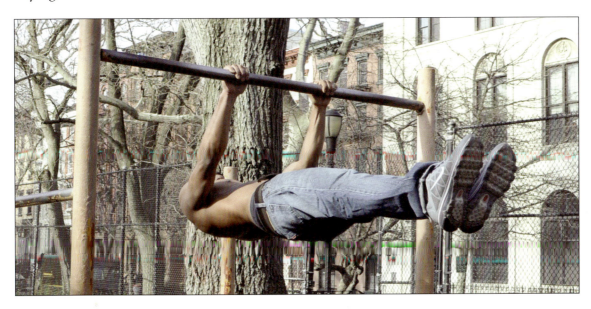

Tuck Front Lever

The easiest variation on the front lever is the tuck front lever. Hang from a pull-up bar and squeeze your legs into your chest while rolling your hips back until your torso is parallel to the ground. Try to stay up and hold this position for as long as you can.

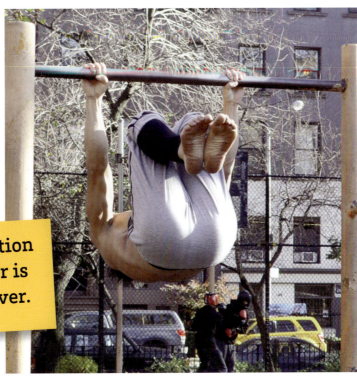

> The easiest variation on the front lever is the tuck front lever.

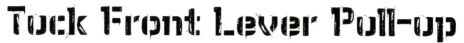

Tuck Front Lever Pull-up

Once you can perform the tuck front lever for ten seconds or more, you can attempt the tuck front lever pull-up. It's best to do these while hanging beneath a pair of parallel bars like you would use for a dip. With your body hanging below the bars, pull your knees into your chest and raise your hips into the tucked front lever position. Make sure you keep your hips up as you pull yourself up between the bars. You can think of this as an advanced version of an Australian pull-up.

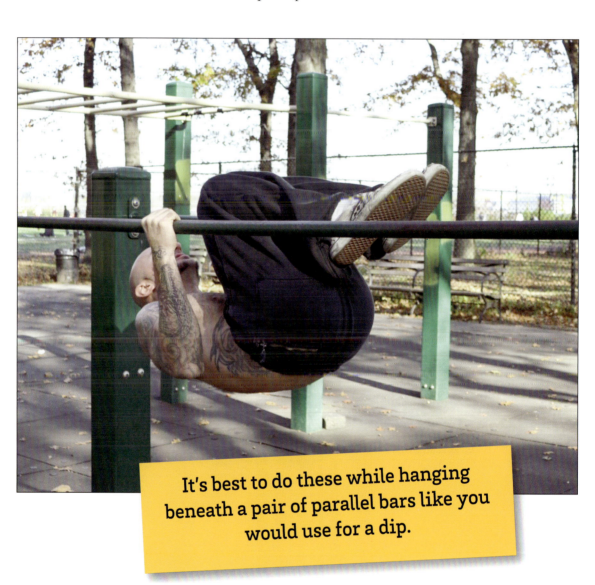

It's best to do these while hanging beneath a pair of parallel bars like you would use for a dip.

Half-Tuck Front Lever

The next step after the tuck front lever is to extend one leg straight. Everything else is more or less the same. You can try pull-ups like this as well once you can get 10 clean tuck front lever pull-ups.

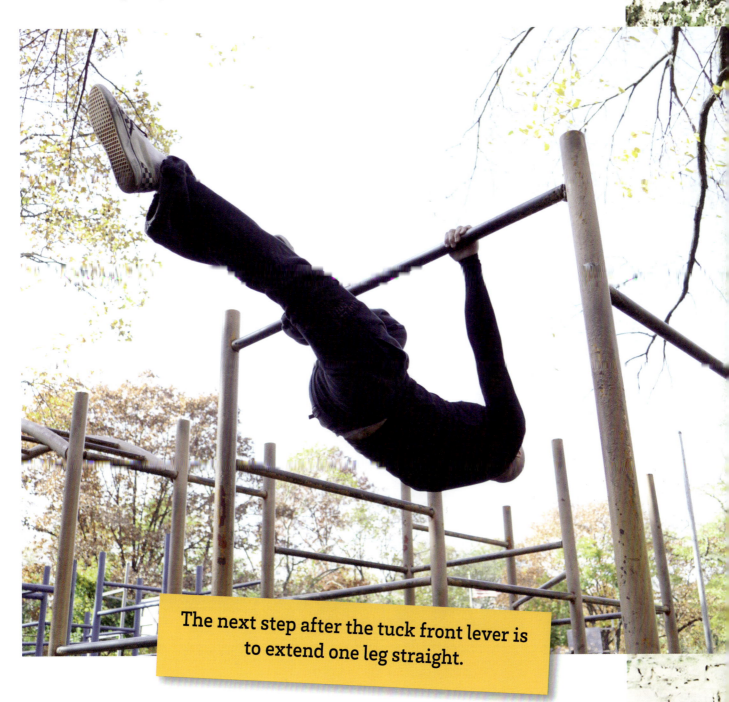

The next step after the tuck front lever is to extend one leg straight.

Straddle Front Lever

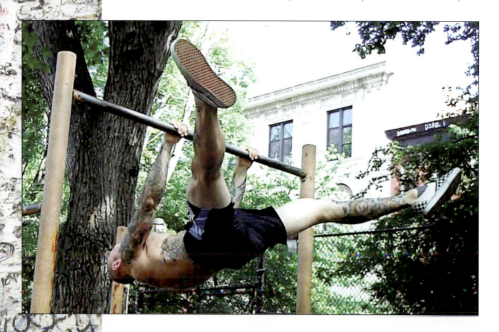

By opening your legs during a front lever, you're not only changing the balance, you're also shortening the lever, both of which make this move slightly easier than a full front lever (though still more difficult than the tuck or half-tuck lever). You'll need better than average hip mobility to pull off a decent straddle front lever, so make sure you're stretching regularly.

Counter-weights

As you get stronger, a common way to make most exercises more challenging is to add weight. The front lever is one of those rare exercises that can actually be made a bit *easier* by adding weight. Wearing a light backpack (around 5-10% of your bodyweight), can actually help you balance in this position. It also looks really cool!

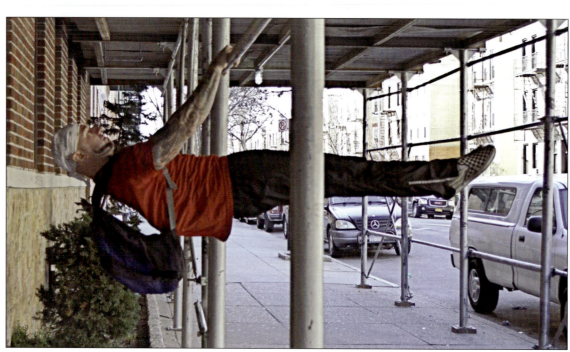

Front Levers for Reps

When building up to a front lever hold, performing front levers for reps from a hanging position can be a very useful tool. Keep your whole body tight as you use your lats to pull your body into the lever position, then lower back down to a dead hang and repeat.

When your form breaks down, switch to hanging leg raises. This can make for a very difficult super-set.

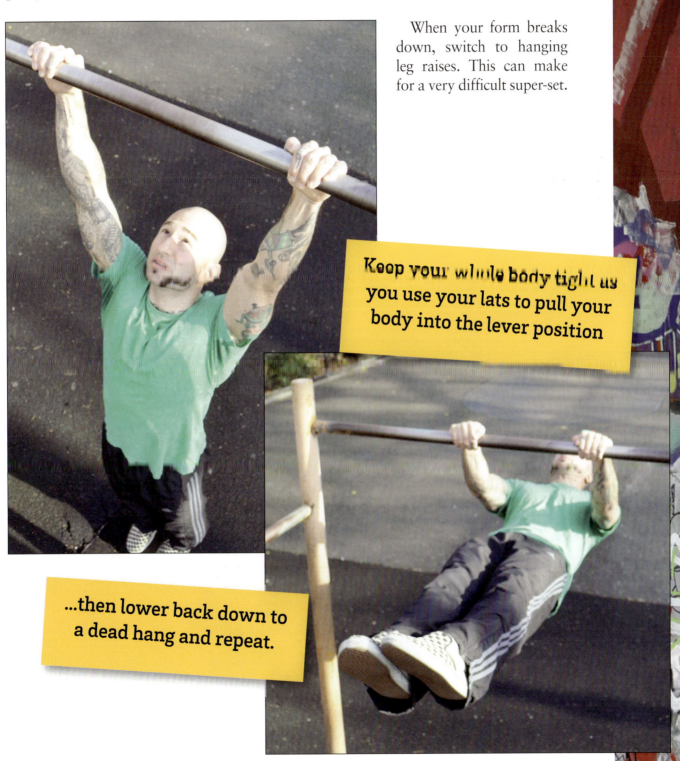

Keep your whole body tight as you use your lats to pull your body into the lever position

...then lower back down to a dead hang and repeat.

Front Lever to Muscle-up

The front lever to muscle-up is a great way to work towards improving your front lever hold, as well as a bad-ass move in its own right. It's easier to do the muscle-up first, then lower yourself into the lever, maintaining total body tension the whole time. Hold the lever position, then pull yourself back over the bar and repeat. Try using a false grip for this maneuver.

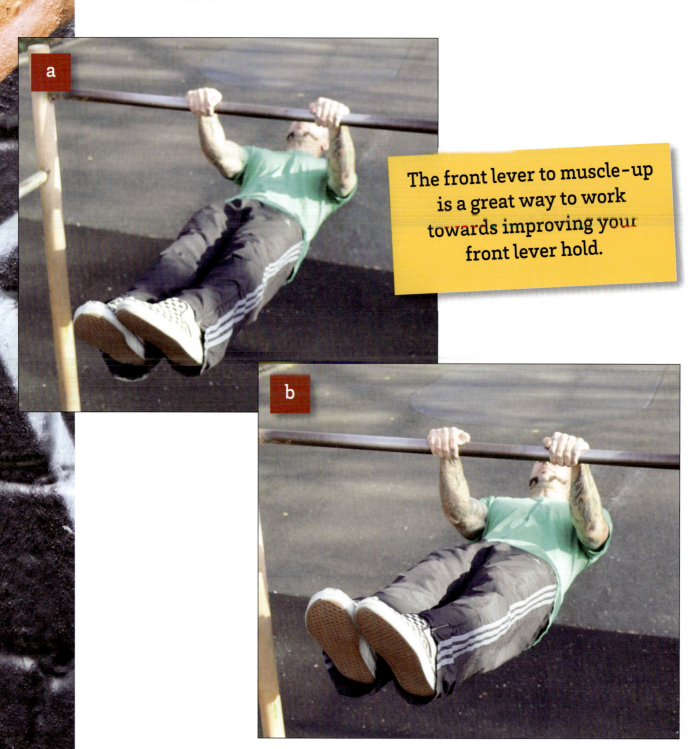

> The front lever to muscle-up is a great way to work towards improving your front lever hold.

Raising the Bar

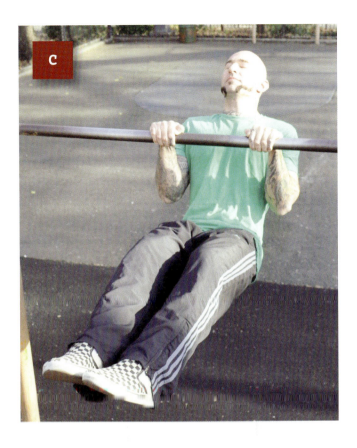

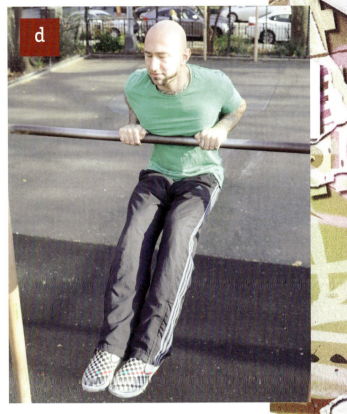

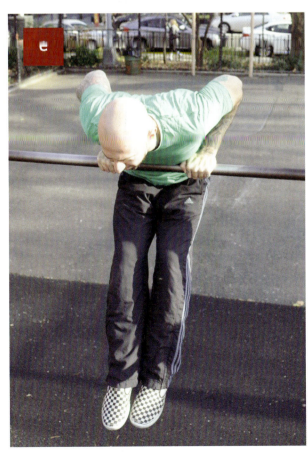

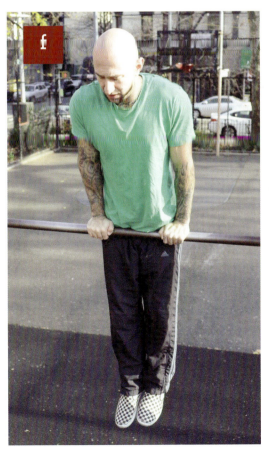

One Arm Lever

Though rarely seen, a one arm front lever is a very advanced variation that is within the spectrum of possibility for someone who is willing to work for it. Likewise, I have seen the back lever performed with just one arm as well. When attempting these variations, keep in mind that the body will need to rotate a bit in order to find balance. I'd give you more advice, but I'm still working on it myself!

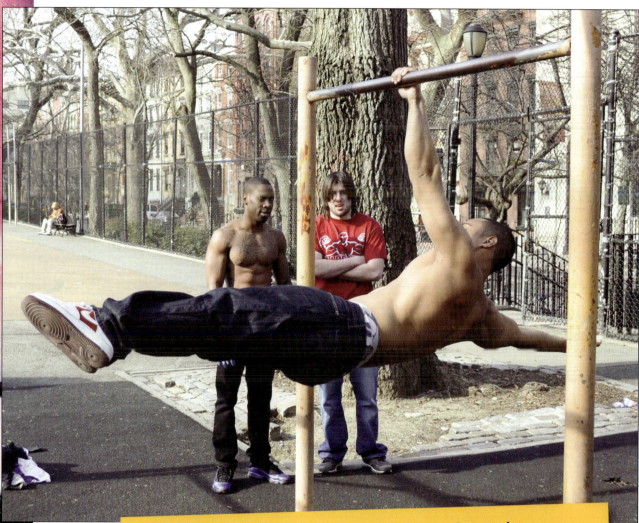

Though rarely seen, a one arm front lever is a very advanced variation that is within the spectrum of possibility for someone who is willing to work for it.

Practice and Progress

While some people will get the elbow lever quickly, working your way up to a front lever hold can take a very long time. Be patient and gradually build to several seconds on each step before moving onto the next one. If you find yourself getting stagnant in your progress, take a break from lever training while you continue to work the basics then come back to it after a few weeks. In the big picture, a little time off from challenging skills like these can sometimes give you renewed focus.

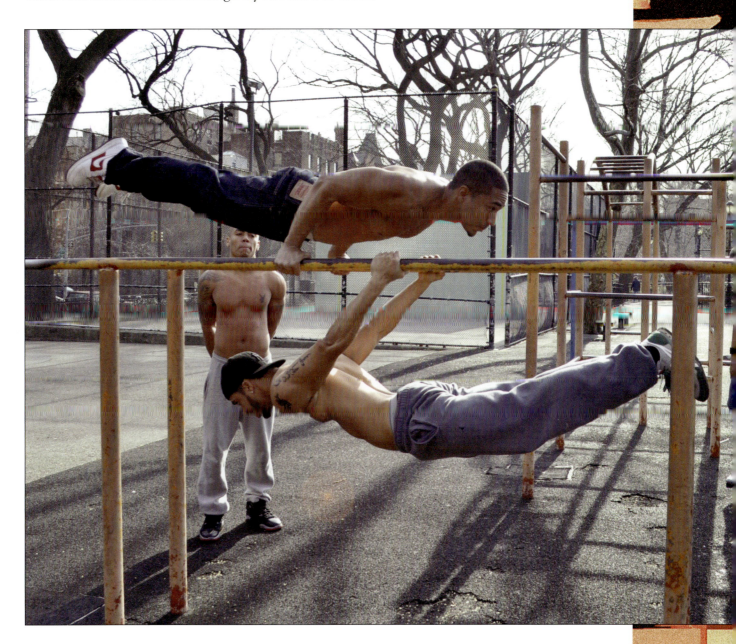

Raising the Bar

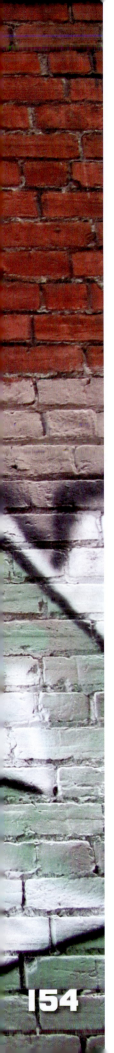
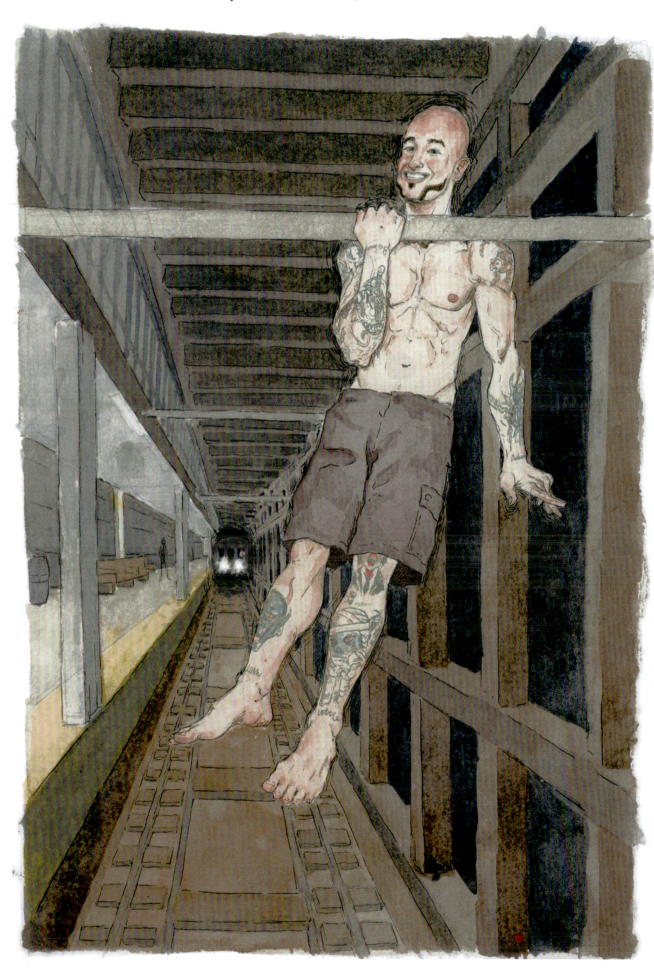

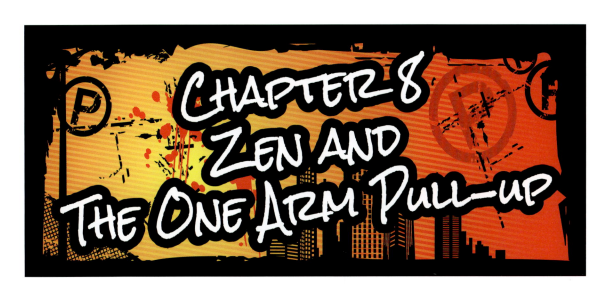

CHAPTER 8
ZEN AND THE ONE ARM PULL-UP

"Strength does not come from
physical capacity.
It comes from an indomitable will"
—Gandhi

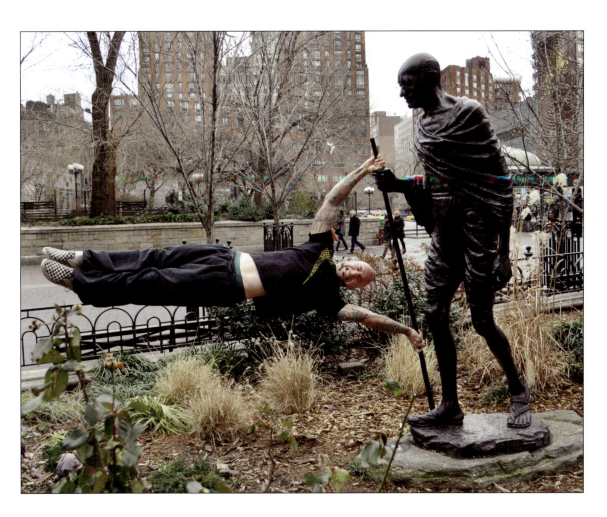

RAISING THE BAR

When I was first starting out as a trainer, I remember having a conversation with a client about whether or not a one arm pull-up was possible. We wound up concluding that the only way it could be done was with the other hand holding the wrist of the primary arm. I often look back and laugh about that conversation now. Boy were we wrong!

Of course, most of the time when you hear someone speak of their ability to do a one arm pull-up, what they are actually bragging about is just that (more of what you might call a one-*handed* pull-up). Let's be clear right off the jump that, while a somewhat impressive feat on it's own, this is not a true one arm pull-up. In fact, anyone who can do about ten pull-ups and has decent grip strength will be able to pop off a couple of one handed pull-ups without much trouble.

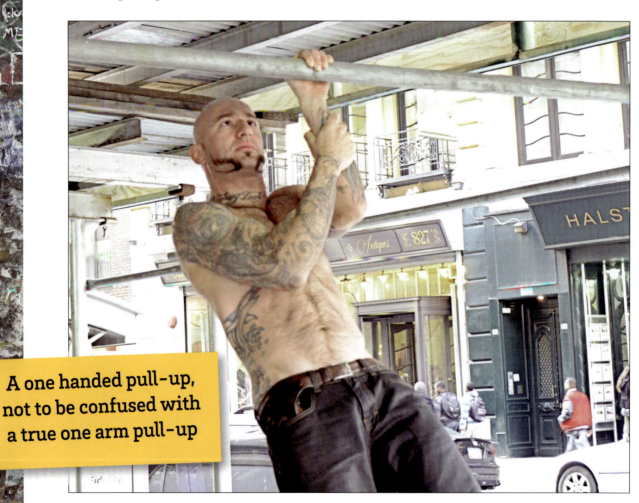

A one handed pull-up, not to be confused with a true one arm pull-up

I'll never forget the first time I saw someone do a legit one arm pull-up. It was in Tompkins Square Park (of course!) in the summer of 2007. Though I'd never seen one before that day, I'm sure people have been doing them for a long, long time - just not that many people. The statistic I've often heard is that only one in 100,000 men can perform this feat, but I think it's within the potential of any man to do at least one rep. The problem is that most people lack the dedication and patience to ever get close to their full potential.

The Humbling

The one arm pull-up is the single hardest pull-up variation I know. That's why I saved it for the end. A few freaks of nature might be able to pull one of these off without much specific training, but the rest of us are looking at a solid year of dedicated training even once you can do lots of standard pull-ups. Be prepared to fail at this move for a very long time before you get it.

Beginner's Mind

Though I've been training one arm pull-ups on and off for five years, they remain a challenge. Some days I can bang out a couple one arm chin-ups without too much trouble, other days I struggle to get even one decent rep. The one arm pull-up is an elusive enigma that reminds me to keep training hard.

Pull-up or Chin-up

Like we discussed back in Chapter One, a pull-up is done with a pronated (overhand) grip, while a chin-up implies a supinated (underhand) grip. When you do a one arm pull-up, however, there's a certain amount of rotation that's virtually unavoidable. This is why many of the people who can perform this feat will wind up bringing the bar towards the shoulder opposite their pulling arm. For me, the disparity between overhand and underhand grips seems negligible. I've done so many reps of different kinds of pull-ups over years that I may have just evened it out. Besides, when someone is strong enough to pull their chin over the bar with just one arm, they've earned my respect. Nitpicking about their hand position seems pointless.

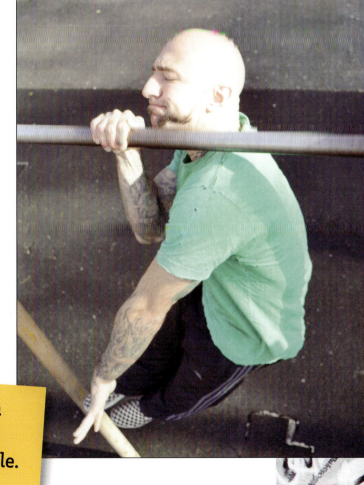

When performing a one arm pull-up, a certain amount of rotation is virtually unavoidable.

Training for a One Arm Pull-up

Only once you can perform *at least* fifteen consecutive dead hang pull-ups should you even consider training for this feat. The one arm pull-up is more advanced than any of the other exercises in this book. It's the ultimate pull-up - that's why it gets it own chapter! Keep that in mind when you begin your journey. It's going to be a long one.

One more word of caution before we begin here; tendinitis is a bitch, so back off if you start to get pain in or around your elbows or shoulders. Rest is a very important part of strength training. Remember that your tendons and other connective tissue also need time to adapt to the demands of the one arm pull-up. I can't stress enough the importance of taking your time with this move. Focus on the process.

One Arm Hangs

Training for a one arm pull-up is a lot like starting over from scratch. In fact, the training is pretty much the same - except you do everything with just one arm! Just like a raw beginner learning to do a two arm pull-up, you'll need to go slowly and manage your expectations. Needless to say, the first thing is to get a solid single arm hang. Try to build to at least 30 seconds (ideally longer) before you move on to the next phase. I also recommend practicing one arm hanging leg raises to get a feel for the stability (or lack thereof). Just like the two arm hangs, remember to pull your shoulder down into your socket and engage your stabilizer muscles.

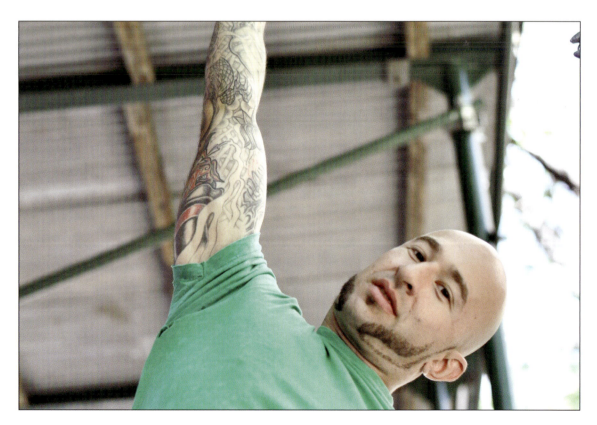

One Arm Flex Hangs

Performing a flex hang with one arm is the next step towards doing a one arm pull-up. Pull yourself up using both arms, then try to stay up while you take one hand away. Squeeze with everything you got! Notice how I am keeping my entire body engaged in the photo to the right.

It's important to note that for all my talk about the negligible disparity between over and underhand grips for well conditioned individuals, the one arm flex hang is best practiced underhand. A supinated grip allows you to keep your arm closer to the middle of your body with your forearm tight against your chest, allowing you better leverage to hold the position. Though I can do an overhand pull-up with one arm, holding the top position for any length of time is much harder. If you can hold an overhand grip one arm flex hang for more than a second or two you must be wickedly strong - I'd love to train with you some time!

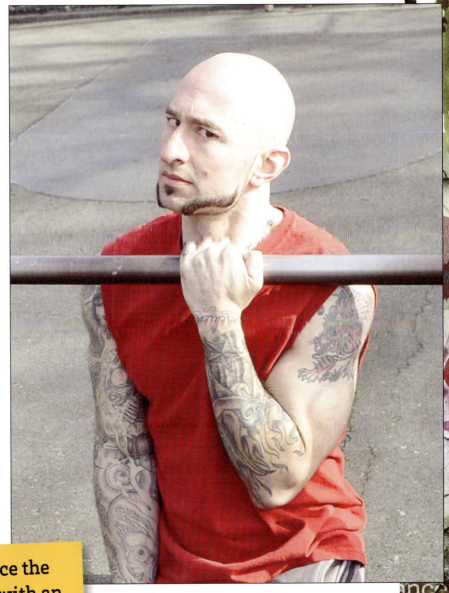

It is best to practice the one arm flex hang with an underhand grip.

One Arm Negatives

We've been over this concept a few times by now. The idea here is to keep your body tight and controlled while slowly lowering yourself down from a one arm flex hang. Be prepared that the first time you try to do a one arm negative you will drop very quickly. When starting out, don't even think of it as a negative, think of it as just trying to keep yourself up. Gravity takes care of the rest. Eventually, try working up to the point where you can make a one arm negative last for ten seconds or longer.

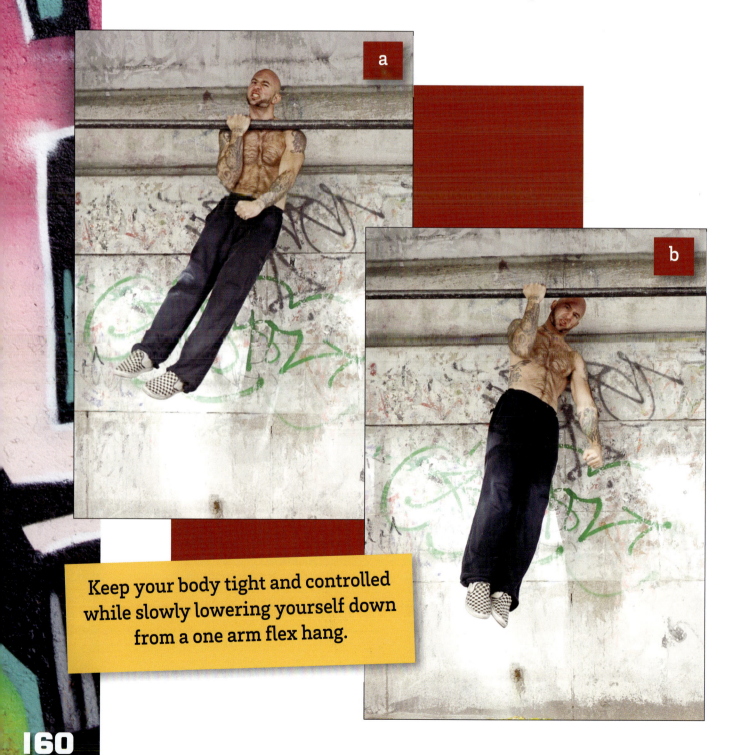

Keep your body tight and controlled while slowly lowering yourself down from a one arm flex hang.

RAISING THE BAR

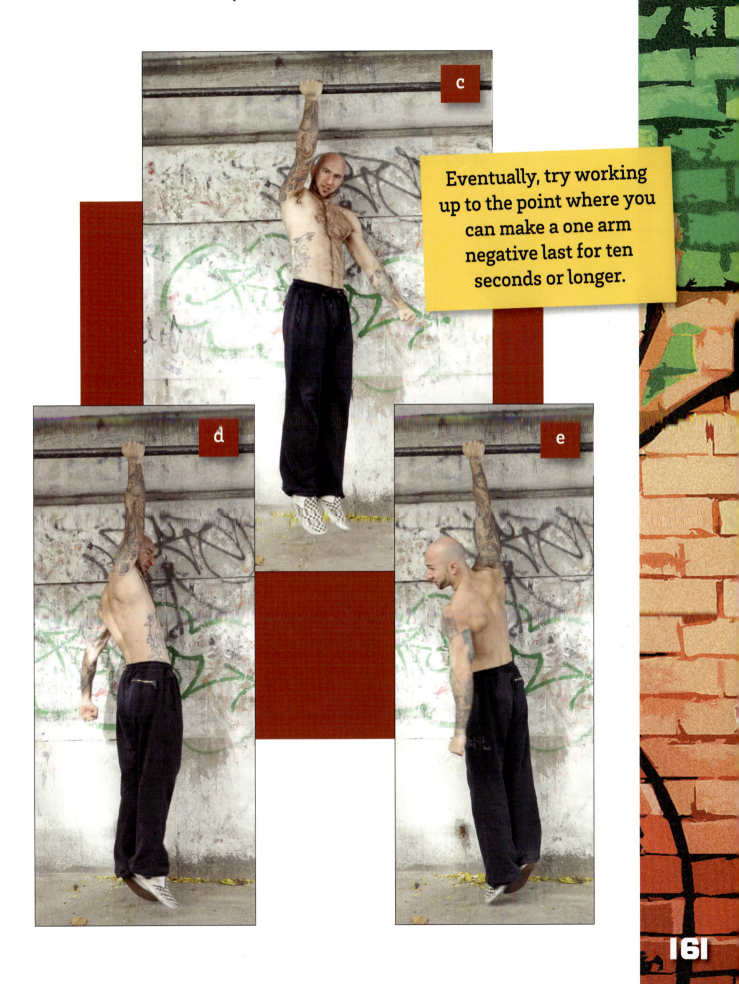

Eventually, try working up to the point where you can make a one arm negative last for ten seconds or longer.

The Self Assist:

Using your free arm to assist your primary arm is a cornerstone of one arm pull-up training. When you're learning to do a regular pull-up, you might need a spotter to assist you, but when you're learning the one arm pull-up, you can be your own spotter! As I mentioned in Chapter Four, an archer pull-up is one type of self assisted one arm pull-up, though there are other ways of achieving the same effect. One way is to practice the one handed pull-up we discussed at the beginning of this chapter.

As with the archer pull-up, when using a one handed pull-up as a means to work towards a true one arm pull-up, try to do as much of the work as possible with your primary arm. Also keep in mind that the further your assisting hand gets from your wrist the less help it can give you. So if you can do more than about 5 reps with your hand on your wrist, try moving your hand down to the bottom of your forearm. When that gets easier, the next step is to place your free hand on your opposite shoulder.

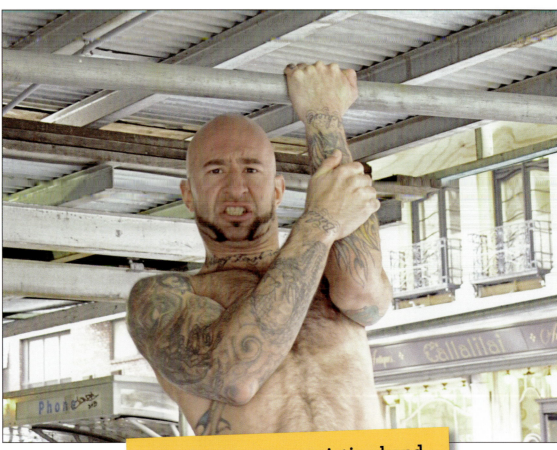

The further your assisting hand gets from your wrist the less help it can give you.

The One Arm Australian Pull-up

This is a nice precursor to the one arm pull-up for the same reason that Australian pull-ups can be a gateway to pull-ups – your feet are on the ground! When attempting a one arm Australian pull-up, concentrate on engaging your abs and your back muscles–focus on using all of your muscles and not just your bicep strength. Remember that when you do a one arm Australian, it's natural for your body to roll a little bit in the direction of your pulling arm. As always, remember to squeeze your whole body tight!

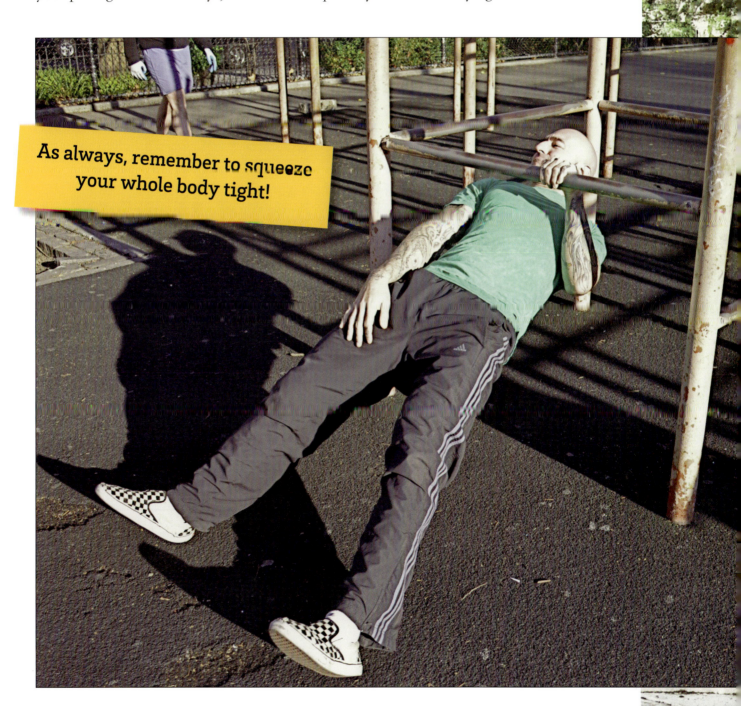

As always, remember to squeeze your whole body tight!

The Other Arm

When you do a one arm pull-up, your opposite arm shouldn't be touching your primary arm in any way, but that doesn't mean it can't help with the movement. Remember our talk about counter balance in Chapter Seven? Reaching your free arm away from your body can change the balance and make the one arm pull-up slightly more manageable. You might find it helpful to reach your legs away as well.

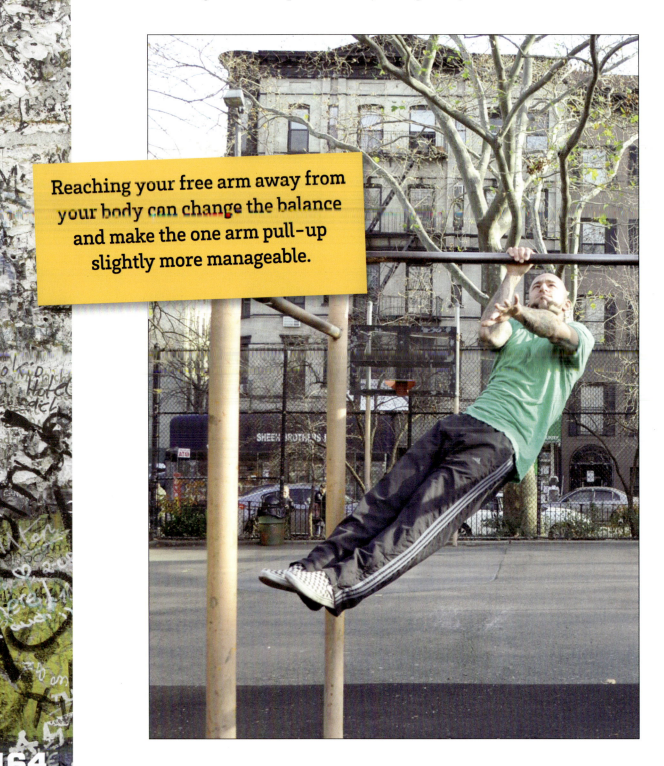

Reaching your free arm away from your body can change the balance and make the one arm pull-up slightly more manageable.

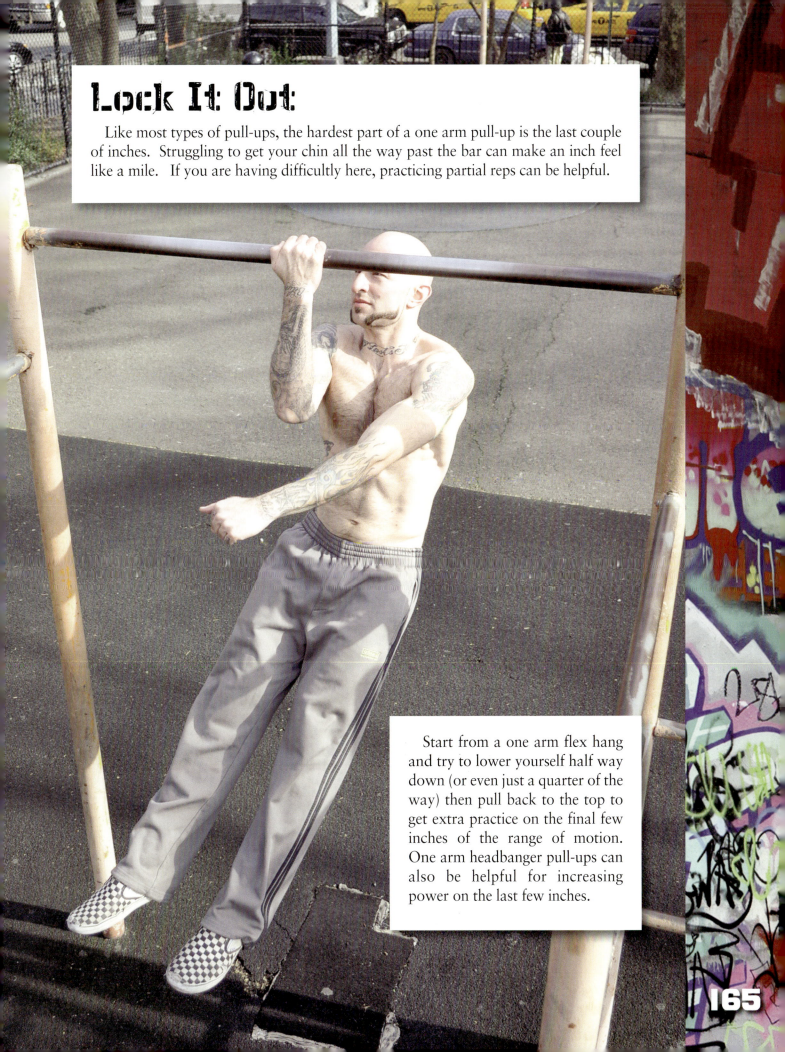

Lock It Out:

Like most types of pull-ups, the hardest part of a one arm pull-up is the last couple of inches. Struggling to get your chin all the way past the bar can make an inch feel like a mile. If you are having difficultly here, practicing partial reps can be helpful.

Start from a one arm flex hang and try to lower yourself half way down (or even just a quarter of the way) then pull back to the top to get extra practice on the final few inches of the range of motion. One arm headbanger pull-ups can also be helpful for increasing power on the last few inches.

Zen and the One Arm Pull-up

While Western thinking tends to get caught up in goals and desires, Zen is all about the present. I tend to agree with this idea of staying in the moment, especially when it comes to training. When training for the one arm pull-up, try to avoid getting too hung up on the end result. Focus on the present and do your flex hangs and negatives with everything you've got - they're very hard exercises in their own right! The journey is the only way to get to the destination, so be there for it or you might miss it altogether. Remember, good things come to those who train.

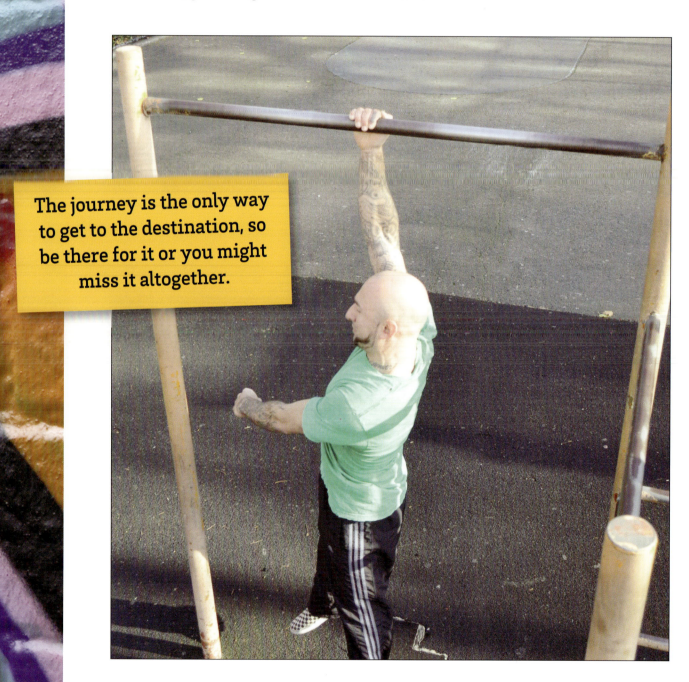

> The journey is the only way to get to the destination, so be there for it or you might miss it altogether.

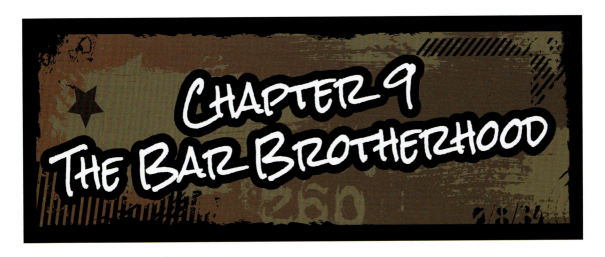

Chapter 9
The Bar Brotherhood

**"With great power
comes great responsibility."
–Spiderman**

While books and websites can be entertaining and educational, there is no substitute for the inspiration that comes from a real flesh and blood training partner. Anyone who has worked out with athletes or had a great personal trainer can tell you that there is no better motivation in the world.

While it's certainly beneficial to train with people who are stronger than you, once you get some experience it can also be worthwhile to have training partners who are less fit that you, so you can inspire them. As the old saying goes, "what goes around comes around." In certain circles, this is referred to as Karma. Besides, seeing a beginner give their all can be very inspiring, regardless of their capabilities.

Of course I charge my personal training clients for my time, but that's just capitalism. Basic economics. Supply and demand. I gave away a lot of free advice over the years to get to the point where people are willing to pay for my time, and I still continue to give away free advice on my blog.

I'm also fortunate to get to train with other inspiring people. I've gotten to work out with some amazing athletes and seen things up close with my own eyes that others can only dream of.

Raising the Bar

I am a lucky guy, but you can be too! If you train with passion and joy, others will want to be around you. This is also a type of Karma. You will bring out the best in each other regardless of who is more fit than the other. Passion is a better attribute in a training partner than strength, though the two are often correlated.

Oh Brother!

My number one training partner is my brother Danny. He and I have been working out together since we were teenagers. We've had many a pull-up contest and even built a backyard pull-up bar together. Over the years we have done a lot to motivate and inspire each other (both on and off the bars).

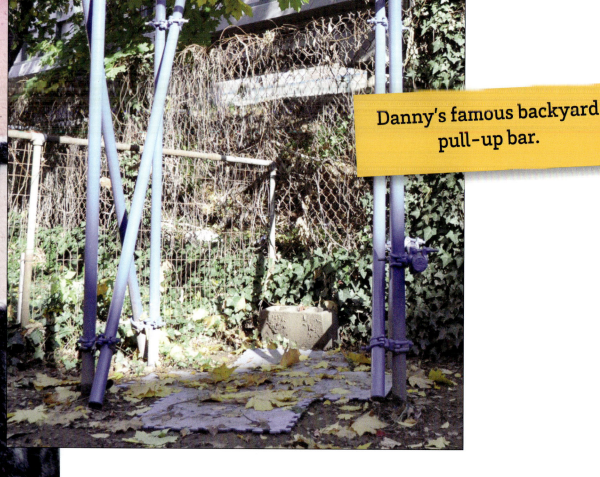

Danny's famous backyard pull-up bar.

Mirror Mirror

Another benefit of a training partner is that you can learn from watching them. Sometimes if Danny and I are working on a new move and he can do it before me, I can then see what mistakes I may be making. Even if I can't learn anything directly from watching him, just seeing it happen right in front of me gets my confidence up to try again! Since Danny and I are actually brothers, we can often act as mirrors for each other to observe and correct our form, but all training partners can do that to some extent. I feel a certain amount of bar-brotherhood with everyone I've trained with over the years who shares the same attitude and love for calisthenics.

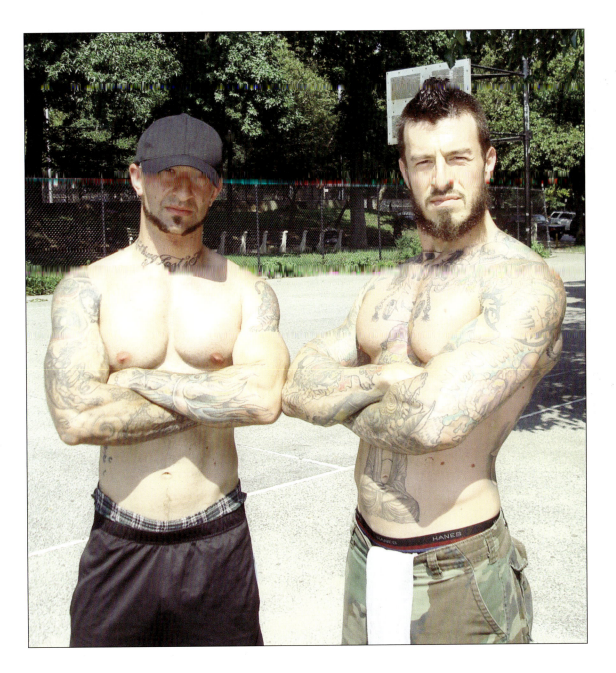

Raising the Bar

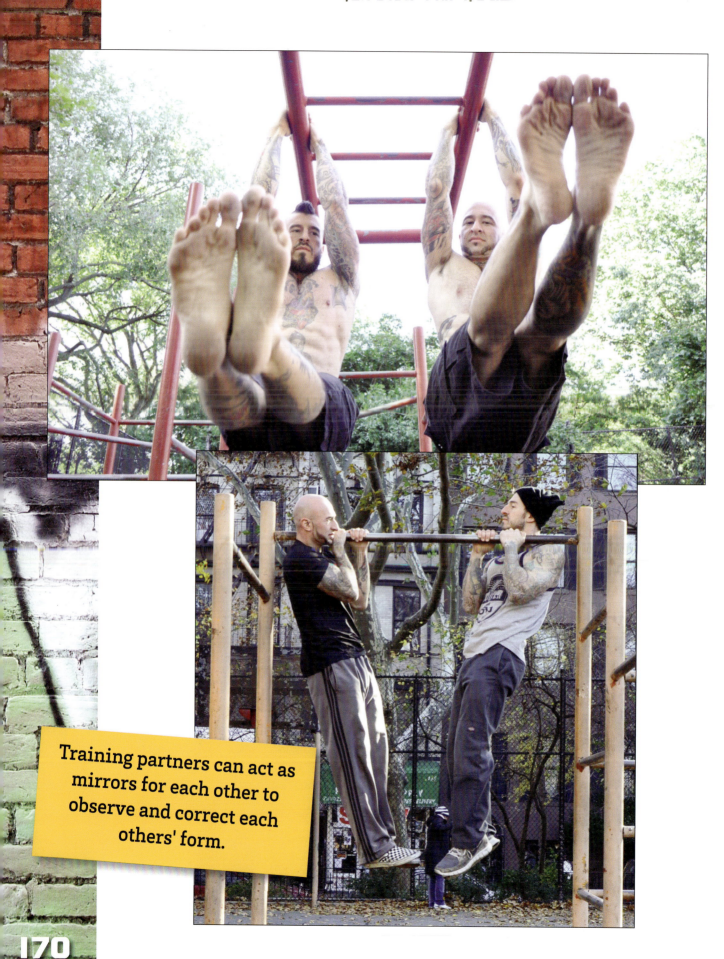

Training partners can act as mirrors for each other to observe and correct each others' form.

Raising the Bar

Teams and Crews

Though people have trained in groups for as long as formal exercise has existed, an interesting thing began happening in the early 2000's. While the Parkour movement was beginning to gather steam in Europe, around NYC's urban parks, calisthenics crews were forming around the pull-up bars. These bar athletes continually challenged one another to up the ante, and through word of mouth, news of these training sessions peaked the interest of local calisthenics enthusiasts. Training sessions would go all day and into the night and demonstrations on scaffolding in Times Square gave tourists something extra to write home about. Pull-up contests like the famous 5B's Pull-up Jam at Brooklyn's Lincoln Terrace Park made newspaper headlines and once video footage from these events made it onto the web, an international phenomenon had been sparked!

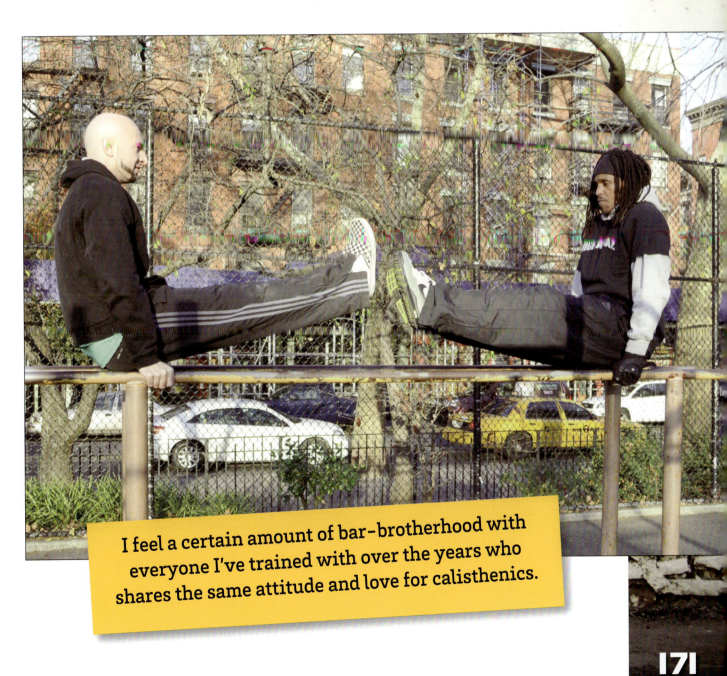

I feel a certain amount of bar-brotherhood with everyone I've trained with over the years who shares the same attitude and love for calisthenics.

Raising the Bar

While it's unclear who the first official team was, the bar calisthenics scene has grown from just a handful of guys at a few local parks into a worldwide phenomenon with new groups popping up in new places every single day. Though rivalries have gotten heated at times, the community as a whole flourishes due to the overwhelming amount of positivity and shared love for the simple beauty of pull-up calisthenics.

As a resident of NYC's East Village for the last several years, I've been lucky enough to be near the heart of one of the calisthenics communities most treasured commodities, Tompkins Square Park. Over the years, I've been lucky enough to train with many of the most noteworthy members of the bar community. Everyone knows that TSP is the place to be if you want to train with world class bar athletes.

Raising the Bar

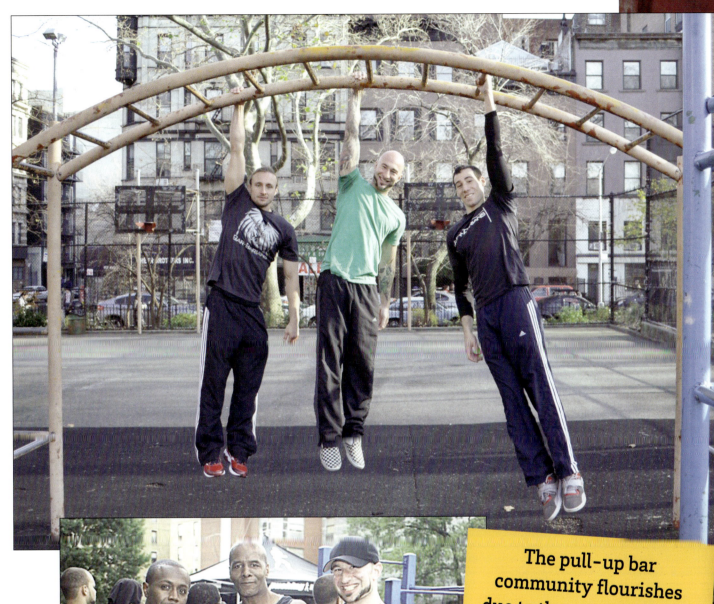

The pull-up bar community flourishes due to the overwhelming amount of positivity and shared love for the simple beauty of calisthenics.

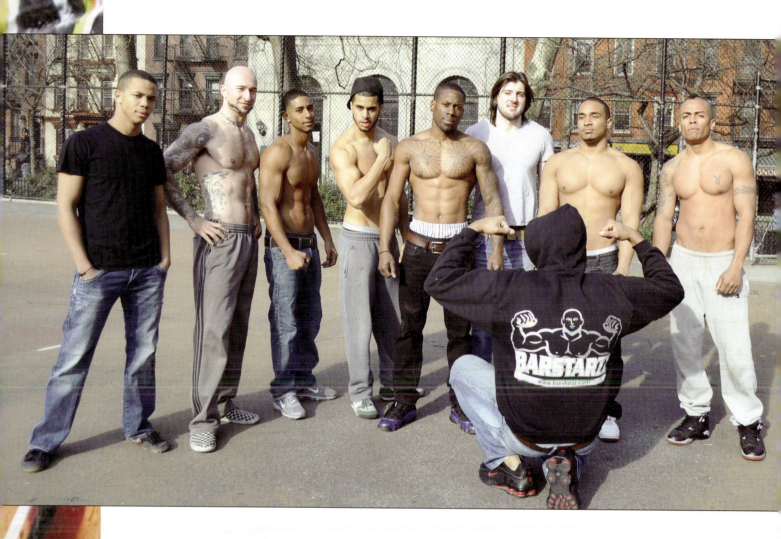

Don't Get Dependent:

While it's great to get a session in with friends when possible, don't get too reliant on them. It's not going to be feasible to train with a partner or trainer every workout; remember that you need to find intrinsic motivation as well.

Simply look inside of yourself and ask, "Why am I doing this?" That answer will be different for different people and the only right answer is the one that keeps you motivated. For me, I couldn't imagine my life without fitness, and pull-ups are my favorite exercise! Physical activity offers a profound opportunity for growth and self discovery. I've learned so much about myself through calisthenics training and I love the journey. The bar never changes, but I certainly do.

RAISING THE BAR

> Simply look inside of yourself and ask, "Why am I doing this?"

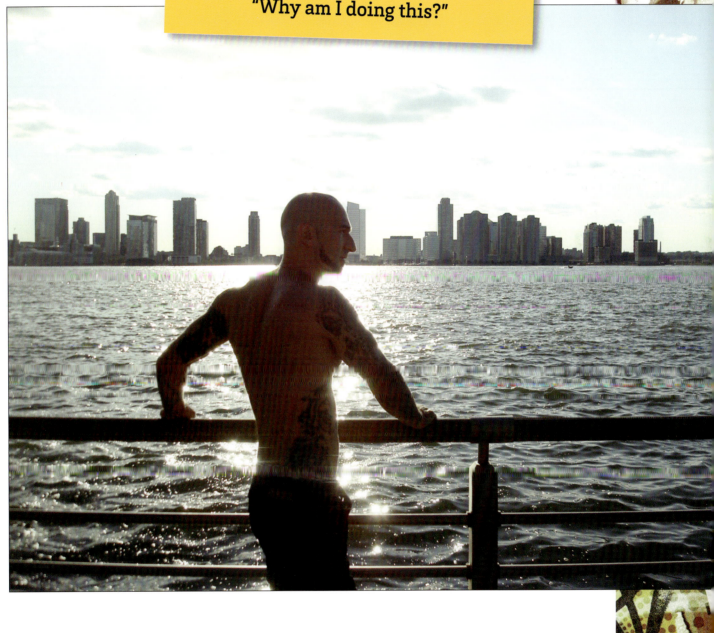

RAISING THE BAR

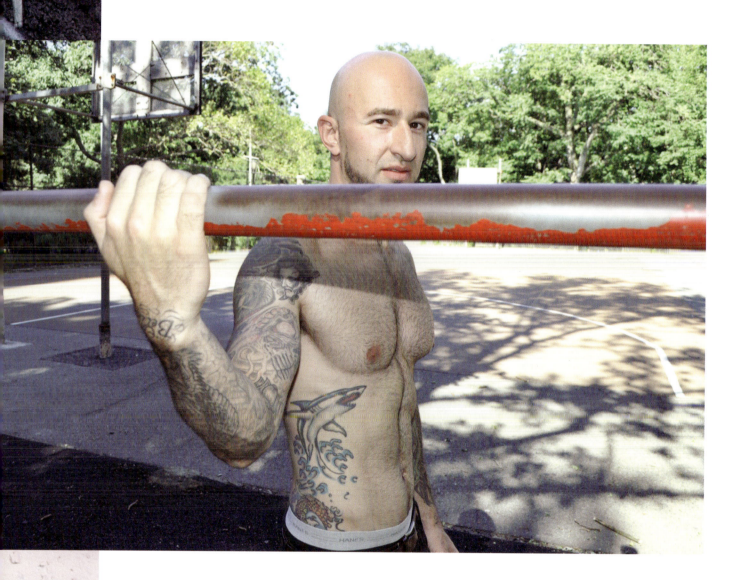

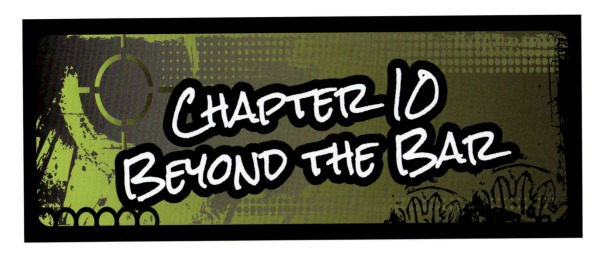

Chapter 10
Beyond the Bar

"It's supposed to be hard.
If it wasn't hard, everyone would do it.
The hard is what makes it great."
–Tom Hanks from *A League of Their Own*

Though there are a few select people who feel proud to be fat, most of us would like to be in better shape. The good news is every one of us can be, the bad news (for some people) is that is requires hard work. Most people spend more time making rationalizations and looking for excuses than they spend looking for solutions. The most common bullshit I hear from people about why they aren't training is that they are too busy or they don't want to pay to use a gym. I can relate to both of these concerns. After all, I'm a pretty busy guy myself and I think gym memberships are usually a rip-off too. Besides, why pay for a gym when you can get fit anywhere?

Any red-blooded man who's walked beneath scaffolding has no doubt been tempted to jump up, grab on and go for it. Those bars are practically begging to be swung around on, hung from or climbed. One of the only things I dislike about my life in NYC is all the construction, but every cloud has a sliver lining. While it can be an eye sore, construction scaffolding is great for doing pull-ups.

RAISING THE BAR

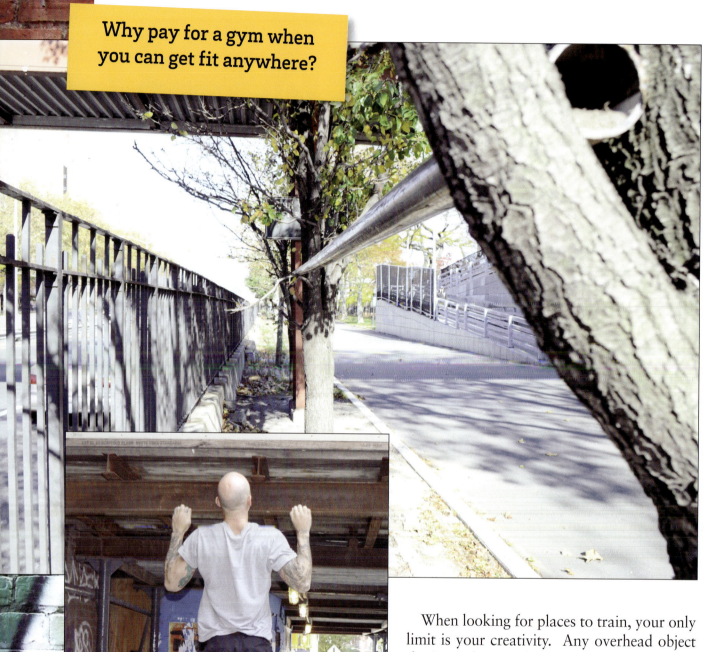

Why pay for a gym when you can get fit anywhere?

When looking for places to train, your only limit is your creativity. Any overhead object that's sturdy enough to support your weight is potentially suitable for pull-ups. Dips can be done in many out-of-the-box scenarios as well. Training on odd objects can sometimes offer unique challenges and benefits. The pull-up shown above offers a unique grip challenge.

While structured workout protocols can be very effective for those who stick to them consistently, you can actually get a lot done without specifically dedicating much extra time (or thought) to your workout. For example, say you pass under a scaffold every morning on your way to work or school, what's to stop you from jumping up and doing just one set on the way there and one set on the way home? This would add less than a minute to your commute each way.

Raising the Bar

Now suppose you could find a place to do some dips during your day-to-day activities and fit a set or two of those in each day. A little bit here and there can add up over time and in a few weeks you would find yourself getting stronger. This technique of "greasing the groove" can be a very effective way to train (more on this in a bit).

I'm sure you can think of plenty of reasons not to train this way. You might feel silly or you might break a sweat in your nice shirt, but guess what? You might actually have some fun!

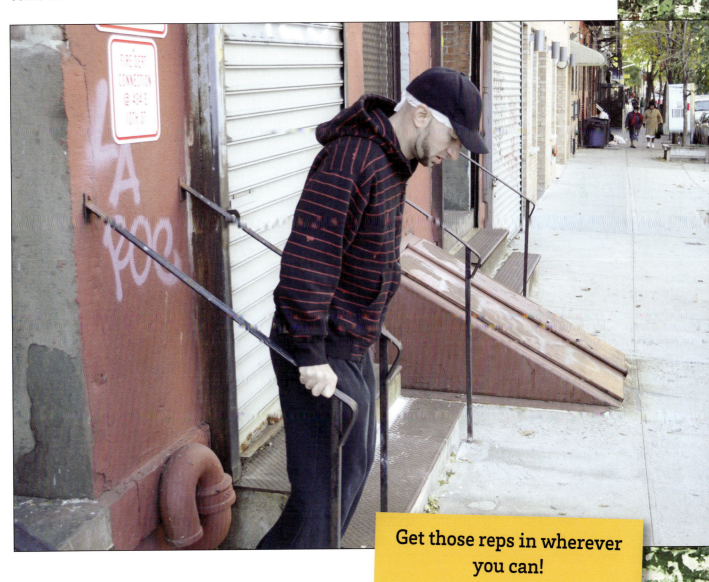

Get those reps in wherever you can!

Freestyle Calisthenics

I want to be perfectly clear that you don't need to do anything more than basic exercises like pull-ups, dips and leg raises to build a strong, muscular upper body. Adding more complicated moves can make your training more interesting, but it won't make you stronger than just training the basics. The world of freestyle calisthenics takes body-weight training out of the realm of exercise and into the performance arena. A lot of the moves I've discussed in this book are as much for showmanship as they are for a workout. Things like muscle-overs won't necessarily make you stronger than regular muscle-ups. However, sometimes focusing on exercise as skill practice can be a great way to divert your focus from the physical rigors of strength training.

With that said, let me restate the first part of that thought: you can get very strong and muscular by just training pull-ups, dips and leg raises. You do not need to train any other movements unless you want to. Don't forget what I said in Chapter One about strength in numbers. Get your reps up on those basic exercises and the strength will be there for the harder ones. Remember as well, that the risk for injury can be higher with some of the more advanced moves and freestyle exercises. Try them at your own risk!

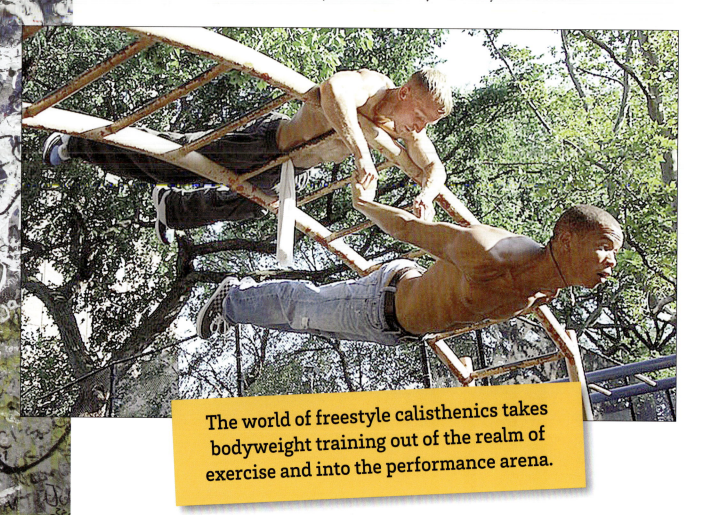

The world of freestyle calisthenics takes bodyweight training out of the realm of exercise and into the performance arena.

Raising the Bar

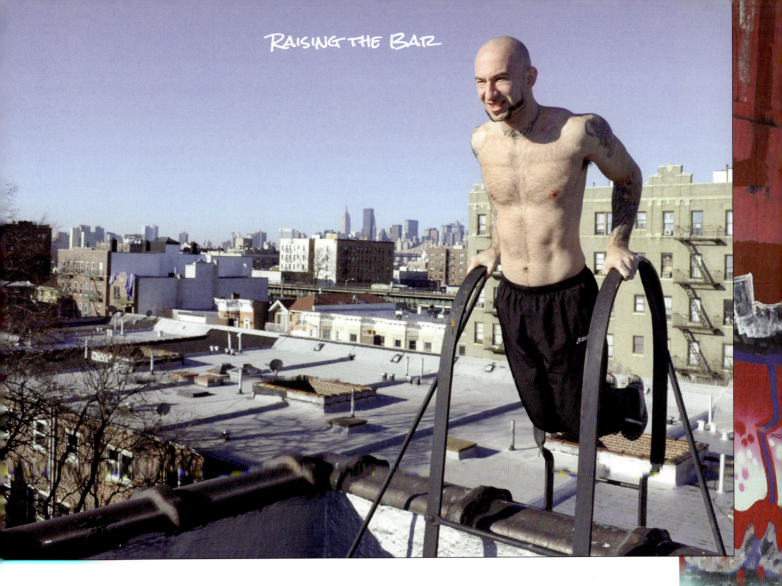

Frequency, Volume and Individual Conditioning

One of the most common questions I get asked is, "can I train calisthenics every day?" The answer is either a "yes" with a "but..." or a "no" followed by an "if..." It's definitely not the same for everyone, but here goes!

Your muscles need rest in order to recover between workouts, but that amount of rest depends on three key factors: frequency, volume and individual conditioning.

Frequency refers to how often you train, volume is how much you do in a given workout and individual conditioning just means how good your individual body is at recovery. That last one comes from a combination of both training and genetic factors. While individual conditioning can be improved dramatically by implementing a fitness regimen, some people are just naturally better at recovery than others. Regardless, people who are training every day need to build to that gradually. Frequency and volume are the two factors you have the most direct control over, but you'll need to experiment to find what works best for you (and is most realistic for your schedule).

Some people (like myself) get great results from exercising every day, while others who feel pressed for time can still make good gains training just three days a week. While I like to exercise daily, I can't go all-out every time or I'll run myself into the ground very quickly. The ratio between frequency and volume is the key to determine how much rest one needs between workouts. As one goes up, the other must go down.

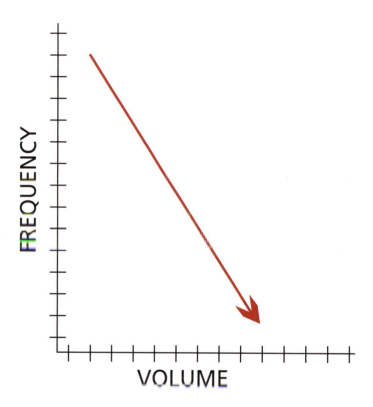

The term "greasing the groove," coined by Pavel Tsatsouline, involves doing just a few reps at a time throughout the day, never working to total fatigue, like the scenario I presented to you before about doing a few scaffold pull-ups on your way around town. A couple reps here and there can add up with this method and great results can be achieved. This is one end of the frequency vs. volume spectrum.

Another underground strength training technique that has been around for a long time and has given many people great results is what's called "German volume training." This method is common in bodybuilding and power-lifting circles. It involves doing many sets of one exercise in one single session. A German volume workout might consist of 100 total reps of a difficult exercise spread out over ten or more consecutive sets, with only a minute or two between each set (who's in for 100 pull-ups?). This type of workout will generally require lots of recovery time as it is extremely taxing on the body. Whereas greasing the groove may help you get strong without ever feeling very sore, German volume training can leave you sore for several days following a workout. Both techniques can be effective, however. There is not always one best method, you just need to make sure you have the right ratio.

A Sore Thing

Some people tend to equate muscle soreness with a good workout, and while that can sometimes be the case, it is not always so. I've had some groundbreaking workouts that left me with minimal soreness and I have had other workouts that left me sore for days even though they didn't do much to improve my fitness. When I ran the NYC Marathon in 2009, my legs were sore as shit for two or three days, but that doesn't mean I should be running a Marathon every time I work out!

As far as I can tell, the only thing that severe muscle soreness reflects is that I did something different than what my body is accustomed (perhaps more volume of the usual exercises or maybe a different modality altogether). For an amateur, this is a good thing. After all, what their body is used to is a whole lotta nothin'. But for someone with a solid training base, being excessively sore may actually prevent you from progressing. Beyond the first few weeks of beginning or restarting a training program, don't put too much stock into whether or not you feel sore.

> When I ran the NYC Marathon in 2009, my legs were sore as shit for two or three days, but that doesn't mean I should be running a Marathon every time I work out!

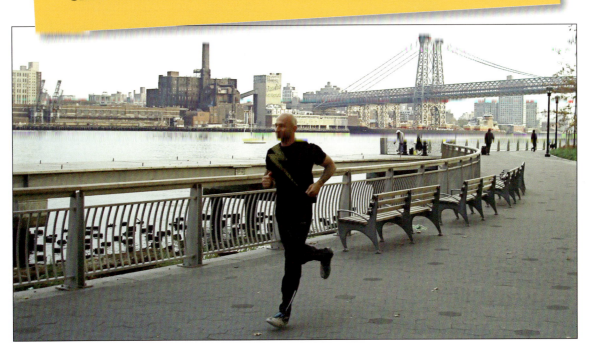

Consistency and Intensity

The number one reason why people don't make progress in their training is a lack of consistency. They train hard for a week or two, then "life gets in the way" and they miss a week or two. This constant one step forward, one step backward approach leaves them standing in the same place year after year.

No matter what type of workout program you choose, you will never get anywhere without consistency. Three times a week is generally the minimum you can train and expect results, but the more often you work out, the better your results are likely to be. Just remember to keep that balance between frequency and volume. Splitting up your training so that you are working on different things on different days is a great way to train without burning yourself out. The most common way to accomplish this is to do all your pulling exercises on one day and all of your pushing exercises on a different day. Like I said in the beginning, you should probably have at least one day for legs in the mix too.

The number two reason people fail to progress is a lack of intensity. You absolutely must be able to push yourself through physical discomfort if you want to build strength and muscle. The funny thing is, your body doesn't really understand the concept of a formal workout. Because of this, it starts telling your brain to stop long before you actually have done enough to affect change in your muscles. The human body hasn't changed much since primitive times, though our lives today are very different. In nature, man needed to conserve his energy. He didn't know when the next meal was coming or what he might have to do to get it. We don't have these concerns in modern society so we can lay it all on the line for our workouts without worrying. Problem is, your mind is still programmed to want to stop as soon as a little fatigue sets in, so you have to be ready for that and prepare yourself to push through. You have to be smarter than your primitive mind.

While the idea of a caveman doing pull-ups seems silly, he may very well have needed to climb a tree to get some berries or to harvest some honey (climbing and pull-ups go hand in hand, by the way). Now suppose as he was climbing that tree his muscles started to burn and his heart started to thump, do you think he would stop? I don't think so! In that situation, stopping could mean starving. How's that for motivation?

Intestinal Fortitude

Several years ago I had an intestinal disease called diverticulitis and required emergency abdominal surgery. Hopefully you are lucky enough to have never experienced such misfortune firsthand. Diverticulitis is generally considered one of the most painful diseases in existence. Brock Lesnar wrote about his experience with diverticulitis in his autobiography, saying it was the toughest opponent he's ever faced in his life, and he was an NCAA champ, a WWE champ and a UFC champ, so he's been in a lot of hard fights. It was certainly far and away the most severe pain I ever felt in my life. When I arrived at the hospital I was writhing in agony. A nurse asked me to look at a chart with the numbers one through ten next to cartoons of different facial expressions. A smiley face was next to the number one, but the expressions grew more and more distressed as the numbers increased. Then the nurse asked me which cartoon I felt like. "Ten!" I cried.

Sometimes I think about that day when I am struggling through a difficult workout. Having lived through my ordeal in the ER, I feel more confident that I can survive the most brutal physical training. The worst discomfort I ever felt while training is maybe a six or seven on the smiley-face scale. I think most people don't know what a ten really feels like. People have gotten coddled too much. Life's gotten easy, but fitness will always require work.

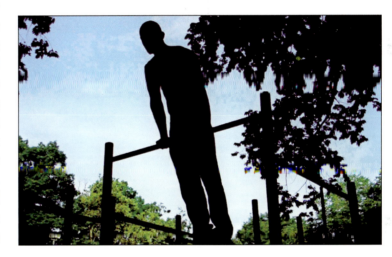

When I say intensity is a factor in your training, I'm talking about what our old friend Tom Hanks was talking about in that quote I mentioned at the start of this chapter. If you aren't willing to suffer for your passion, do not expect to achieve greatness. The bar doesn't care who you are or where you come from. It doesn't care if you are rich or poor. What matters is how much you are willing to endure. So ask yourself...

How bad do you want it?

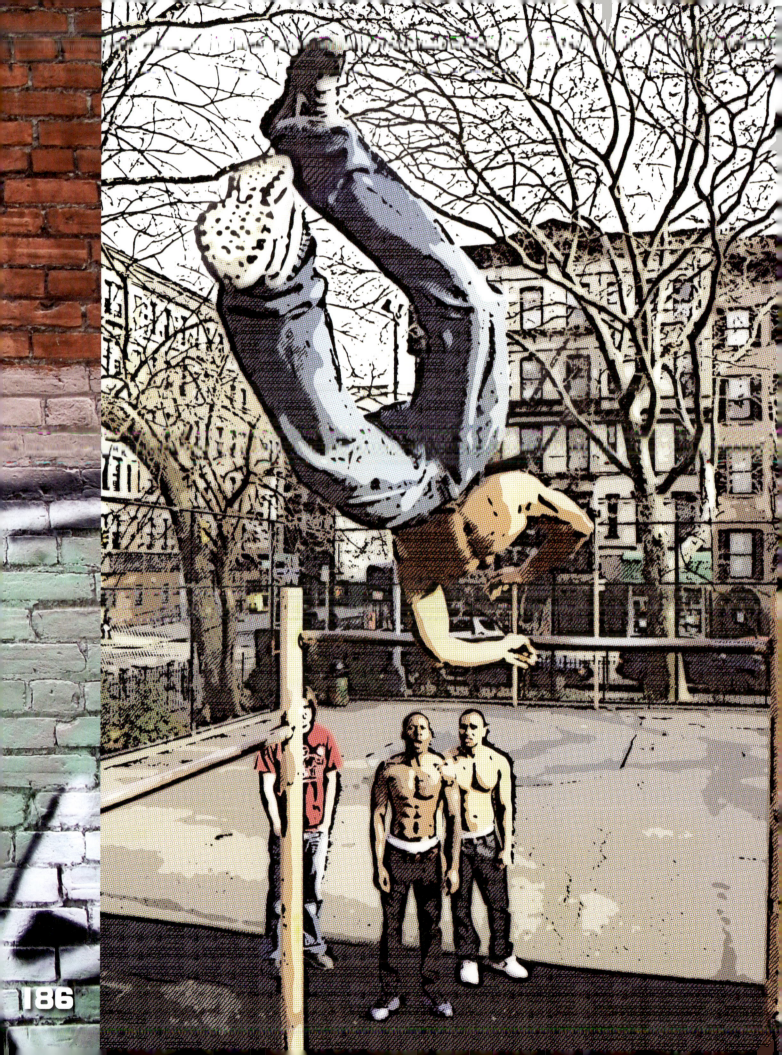

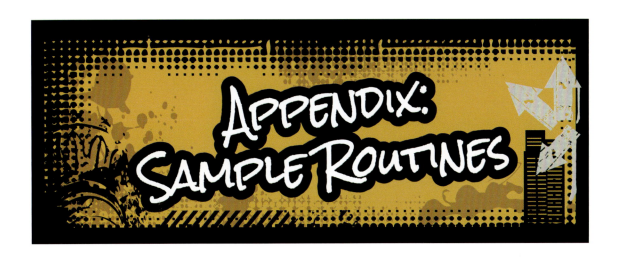

Make Your Own Workout:

There really are no excuses to be weak. No gym membership - no problem. Pressed for time? An intense workout can be done in 20 minutes or less, and Intensity matters more than duration. One of the beautiful things about life is that we all get to create our own destiny. A great body is yours for the taking. If you want it, go get it - it's yours. If you don't, I have no sympathy for you.

I've written the following progressions for people who may be new to bar training to help with program design. Those of you with some experience can feel free to jump in and begin at whichever level you feel is appropriate. Each exercise should be performed for 3-5 sets of up to 10 reps. For exercises that are performed as isometric holds, count every 2 seconds as 1 rep. When you can do the given exercises for 3 sets of 5-10 reps (or 20-30 seconds for the holds), move on to the next level. If you are between levels, feel free to combine aspects of both to fit your needs. Remember, this is a make your own workout!

Novices should begin at level one.

Level 1

Low bar dip
Australian pull-up
Dead hang (overhand)
Flex hang (underhand)
Negative chin-up
Crow pose

Level 2

Parallel bar dip (or perpendicular bar dip)
Chin-up
Overhand flex hang
Hanging knee raise
Elbow lever

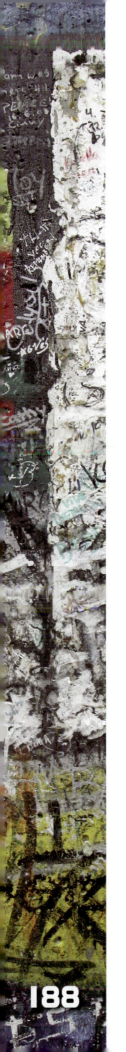

Level 3

Pull-up
Handstand
Pike push-up
Full hanging leg raise, Skin the cat or Rollover
Beginning muscle-up training:
Plyo-pullup/kipping pull-up
Self assisted muscle-up
Tuck back lever/front lever

Level 4

Muscle-up
Handstand push-up
One arm elbow lever
Korean dip
Back lever
Half tuck or straddle front lever
One arm hang, flex hang, negative, etc.

Level 5

One arm hanging leg raise
Front lever
Freestanding handstand push-up
X-muscleup, 360 Muscle-up, etc
One arm pull-up

My Favorite Workouts

Lots of people love my concept of designing your own workout, but others are always asking for specific routines, so here are a few of my favorites. They don't take very long and they will thoroughly work your upper body. As these are pretty intense workouts, I recommend resting on the following day.

The Eliminator

This is a full upper body workout for the advanced trainee. You can do this as a circuit or one exercise at a time. (You may choose to sub pike presses for handstand push-ups.)

Warm-up:

Shoulder rollouts 3 sets of 10 front to back, take your time

The Workout:

3 sets of each exercise,
  1 minute rest in between sets
First two sets: 10 reps or failure (whichever happens first)
Third set: Failure

The Exercises:

Handstand push-ups
Muscle-ups
Pull-ups

If you've got anything left, do another set of each exercise to failure.

Back to Basics

Perform each of the following exercises for 5 sets of 10 reps. You can do this as either a circuit workout or by doing the 5 sets of each exercise in succession with a minute of rest in between. Use a harder variation of each exercise if you can get through this easily (for example: plyo pull-ups in place of pull-ups).

The Exercises:

Pull-ups
Dips
Hanging Knee Raises

Pull-up Madness

2 sets of each exercise - ten reps or til failure (whichever happens first). I recommend consecutive sets of each exercise in order with a minute or two of rest in between.

The Exercises:

Pull-ups
Commando pull-ups
Archer pull-ups
Headbanger pull-ups
Decline Australian pull-ups

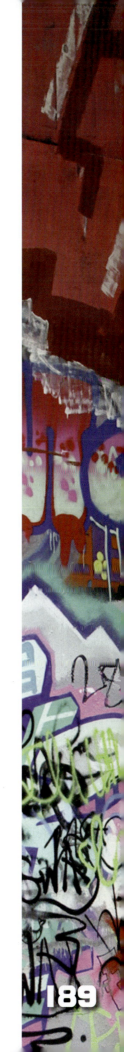

Assessing Your Strength

The tables below offer guidelines by which to asses your strength on the three main exercises discussed in this book: pull-ups, dips and hanging leg raises. The numbers refer to consecutive reps performed in one set without coming down from the bar(s). You can stop for a breath if you need to, but don't let go or the set is over. I recommend testing yourself once every few weeks or months, always emphasizing form over quantity.

MEN

	Pull-ups	Parallel Dips	Hanging Leg Raises
Novice	<5	<5	<1
Beginner	5-10	5-14	1-4
Intermediate	11-17	15-30	5-10
Advanced	18-25	31-45	11-15
Elite	26 & up	46 & up	16 & up

WOMEN

	Pull-ups	Parallel Dips	Hanging Leg Raises
Novice	<1	<1	<1
Beginner	1-2	1-3	1-4
Intermediate	3-6	4-8	5-10
Advanced	7-10	9-14	11-15
Elite	11 & up	15 & up	16 & up

Acknowledgements

First off, thanks to my parents, Carl and Rosalie and my brothers Danny and Jesse for all the love, support and inspiration over the last 32 years. I am blessed to have such an amazing family.

Thank you to Colleen Leung, whose photos are as much a part of this book as I am. Colleen went above and beyond for this project, taking thousands of photos over the course of several months. She and I were very picky about which made it into the book. The ones in here are the best of the best.

Thanks to Paul Wade for writing such an awesome foreword for this book, and for all the exposure he's given me in the bodyweight strength community through appearing in his latest book, **Convict Conditioning 2**. (Buy it if you haven't yet!)

Thanks to John Du Cane for teaching me how to spell "foreword" and for everything else he did to help make this book possible. John is a class act - it's been a pleasure working with him and the rest of the team at Dragon Door.

Thanks to "Big D" Derek Brigham for doing such an amazing job with the book design and cover. Derek's ability to realize my vision while putting in his own signature style has made this book look even better than I ever thought possible.

Thanks to Daniel Lucas, Keith Paine, Antonio Sini and the rest of the team at Nimble Fitness in NYC. These guys have believed in me and supported me from the moment I met them and I am grateful for it.

Of course, a big thank you to all the pull-up bar athletes that inspired me over the years and to everyone who spreads positivity in the bar community.

Last but not least, thanks to all my other friends, family, coworkers and clients who have supported me and brought positivity into my world. This book wouldn't have been possible without each and every one of you.

We're Working Out!

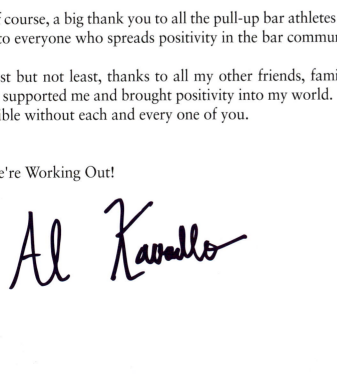

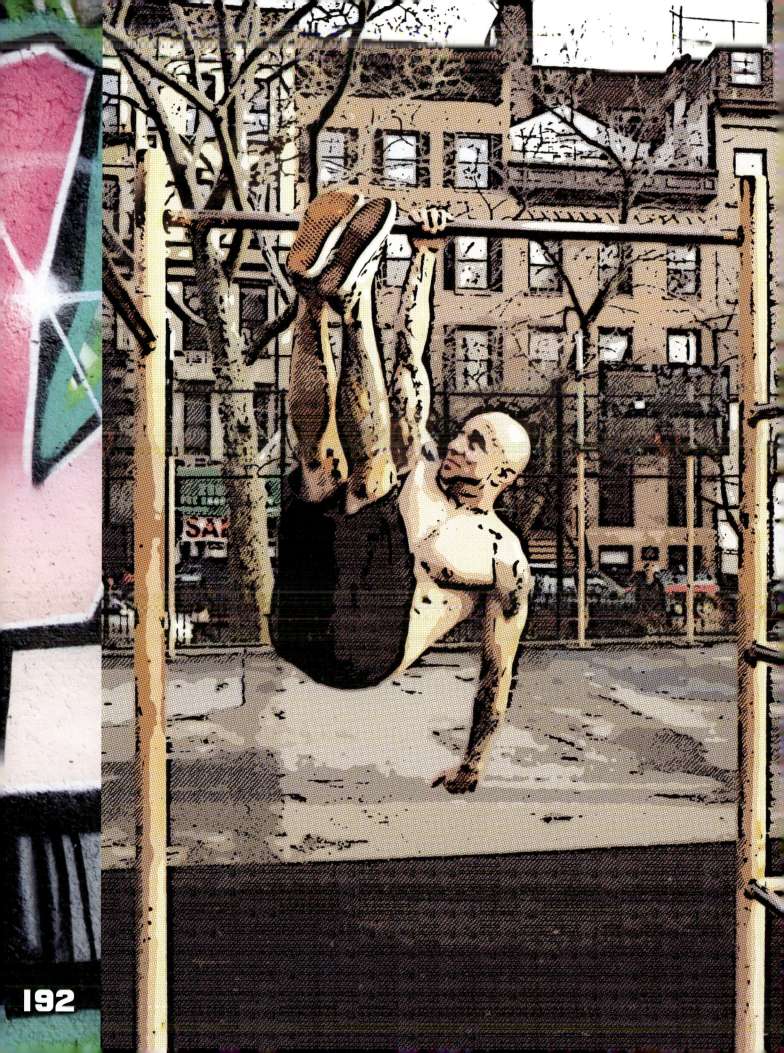

ABOUT THE AUTHOR

Al Kavadlo, CSCS is one of New York City's most passionate and successful personal trainers. A fixture in the ever changing fitness scene, Al has worked with all types of clients, including athletes, models and even an Olympic medalist. Al is recognized worldwide for his amazing bodyweight feats of strength, and his blog (**www.AlKavadlo.com**) has become one of the most popular online resources for information about bodyweight strength training and calisthenics. Al also shares his unique perspective and exercise philosophy in his first book, *We're Working Out! A Zen Approach to Everyday Fitness*.

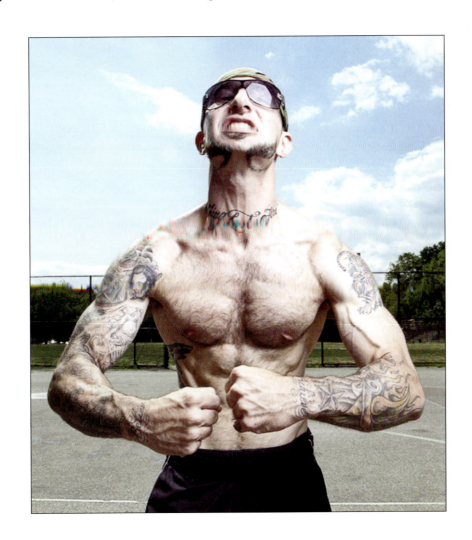

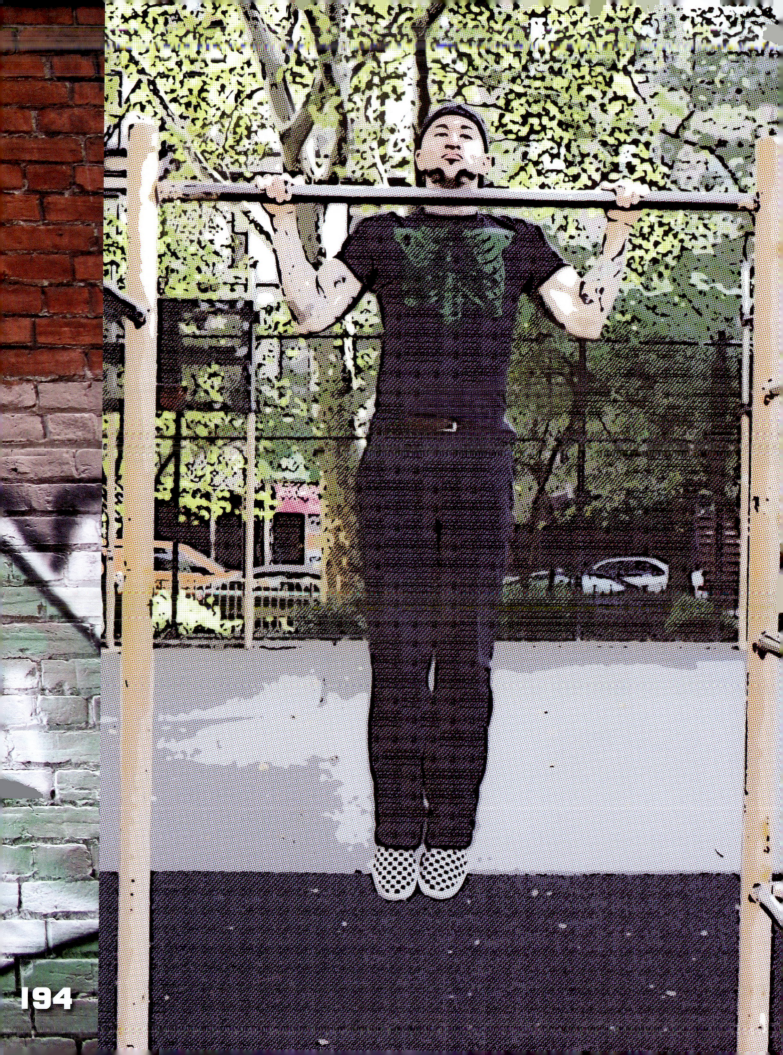

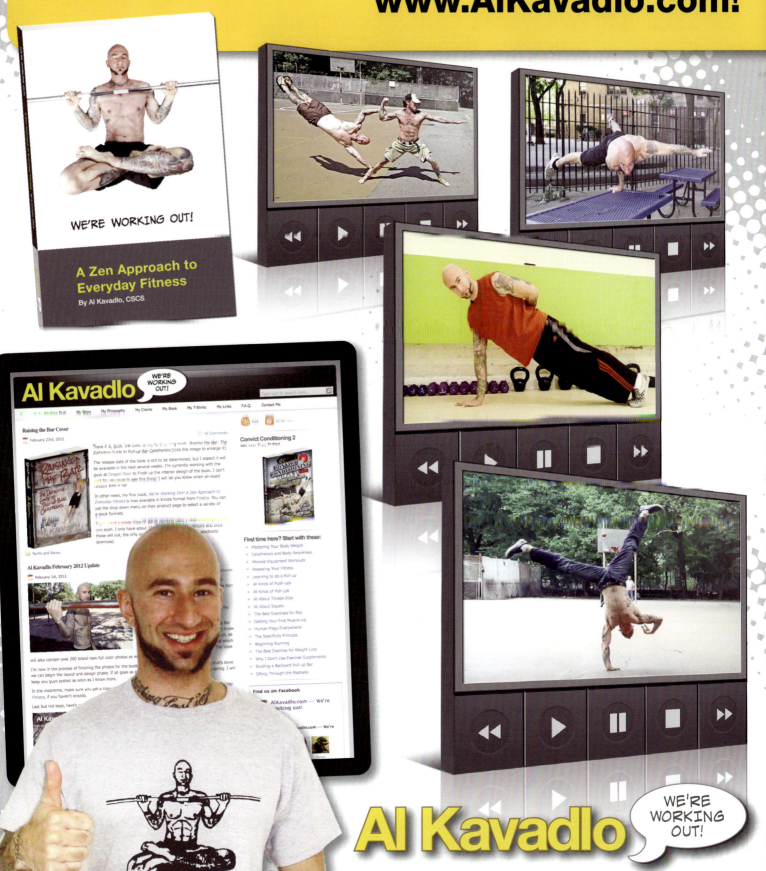

How Do YOU Stack Up Against These 6 Signs of a TRUE Physical Specimen?

According to Paul Wade's *Convict Conditioning* you earn the right to call yourself a "true physical specimen" if you can perform the following:

✓ 1. AT LEAST one set of 5 one-arm pushups each side—with the ELITE goal of 100 sets each side

✓ 2. AT LEAST one set of 5 one-leg squats each side—with the ELITE goal of 2 sets of 50 each side

✓ 3. AT LEAST one set of 1 one-arm pullups each side—with the ELITE goal of 2 sets of 6 each side

✓ 4. AT LEAST one set of 5 hanging straight leg raises—with the ELITE goal of 2 sets of 30

✓ 5. AT LEAST one set of 1 stand-to-stand bridges—with the ELITE goal of 2 sets of 30

✓ 6. AT LEAST one set of 1 one-arm handstand pushups—with the ELITE goal of 1 set of 5

Well, how DO you stack up?

Chances are that whatever athletic level you have achieved, there are some serious gaps in your OVERALL strength program. Gaps that stop you short of being able to claim status as a truly accomplished strength athlete.

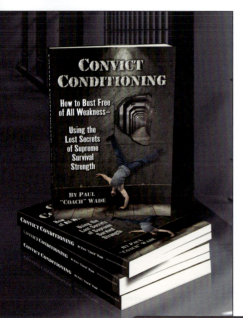

The good news is that—in *Convict Conditioning*—Paul Wade has laid out a brilliant 6-set system of 10 progressions which allows you to master these elite levels.

And you could be starting at almost any age and in almost in any condition...

Paul Wade has given you the keys—ALL the keys you'll ever need— that will open door, after door, after door for you in your quest for supreme physical excellence. Yes, it will be the hardest work you'll ever have to do. And yes, 97% of those who pick up *Convict Conditioning*, frankly, won't have the guts and the fortitude to make it. But if you make it even half-way through **Paul's Progressions**, you'll be stronger than almost anyone you encounter. Ever.

Here's just a small taste of what you'll get with *Convict Conditioning*:

Can you meet these 5 benchmarks of the *truly* powerful?... Page 1

The nature and the art of real strength... Page 2

Why mastery of *progressive calisthenics* is the ultimate secret for building maximum raw strength... Page 2

A dozen one-arm handstand pushups without support—anyone? Anyone?... Page 3

How to rank in a powerlifting championship—*without ever training with weights*... Page 4

Calisthenics as a hardcore strength training technology... Page 9

Spartan "300" calisthenics at the Battle of Thermopolylae... Page 10

How to cultivate the perfect body—the Greek and Roman way... Page 10

The difference between "old school" and "new school" calisthenics... Page 15

The role of prisons in preserving the older systems... Page 16

Strength training as a primary survival strategy... Page 16

The 6 basic benefits of bodyweight training... Pages 22—27

Why calisthenics are the *ultimate* in functional training... Page 23

The value of cultivating *self-movement*—rather than *object-movement*... Page 23

The *real* source of strength—it's not your *muscles*... Page 24

One crucial reason why a lot of convicts deliberately avoid weight-training... Page 24

How to progressively strengthen your joints over a lifetime—and even heal old joint injuries... Page 25

Why "authentic" exercises like pullups are so perfect for strength and power development... Page 25

Bodyweight training for quick physique perfection... Page 26

How to normalize and regulate your body fat levels—with bodyweight training only... Page 27

Why weight-training and the psychology of overeating go hand in hand... Page 27

The best approach for rapidly strengthening your whole body is this... Page 30

This is the most important and revolutionary feature of *Convict Conditioning*... Page 33

A jealously-guarded system for going from puny to powerful—when your life may depend on the speed of your results... Page 33

The 6 "Ultimate" Master Steps—only a handful of athletes in the whole world can correctly perform them all. Can you?... Page 33

How to Forge Armor-Plated Pecs and Steel Triceps... Page 41

Why the pushup is the *ultimate* upper body exercise—and better than the bench press... Page 41

How to effectively bulletproof the vulnerable rotator cuff muscles... Page 42

Order *Convict Conditioning* online: www.dragondoor.com/B41

24 HOURS A DAY ORDER NOW CALL **1·800·899·5111**

196

Observe these 6 important rules for power-packed pushups... Page 42

How basketballs, baseballs and *kissing-the-baby* all translate into greater strength gains... Page 44

How to guarantee steel rod fingers... Page 45

Do you make this stupid mistake with your push ups? This is wrong, wrong, wrong!... Page 45

How to achieve 100 consecutive one-arm pushups each side... Page 64

Going Beyond the One-Arm Pushup... Pages 68—74

Going up!— how to build elevator-cable thighs... Page 75

Where the *real* strength of an athlete lies... Page 75

Most athletic movements rely largely on this attribute... Page 76

The first thing to go as an athlete begins to age—and what you MUST protect... Page 76

THE best way to develop truly powerful, athletic legs... Page 77

The phenomenon of *Lombard's Paradox*—and it contributes to power-packed thighs... Page 78

Why bodyweight squats blow barbell squats away... Page 79

The enormous benefits of mastering the one-leg squat... Page 80

15 secrets to impeccable squatting—for greater power and strength... Pages 81—82

Transform skinny legs into pillars of power, complete with steel cord quads, rock hard glutes and thick, shapely calves... Page 102

How to achieve one hundred perfect consecutive one-leg squats on each leg... Page 102

Going Beyond the One-Leg Squat... Pages 106—112

How to add conditioning, speed, agility and endurance to legs that are already awesome.... Page 107

How to construct a barn door back—and walk with loaded guns... Page 113

Why our culture has failed to give the pullup the respect and attention it deserves... Page 113

Benefits of the pullup—king of back exercises... Page 114

The dormant superpower for muscle growth waiting to be released if you only do this... Page 114

Why pullups are the single best exercise for building melon-sized biceps... Page 115

Why the pullup is THE safest upper back exercise... Page 115

The single most important factor to consider for your grip choice... Page 118

How to earn lats that look like wings and an upper back sprouting muscles like coiled pythons... Page 138

How to be strong enough to rip a bodybuilder's arm off in an arm wrestling match... Page 138

How to take a trip to hell—and steal a Satanic six-pack... Page 149

The 5 absolute truths that define a genuine six-pack from hell... Page 150

This is the REAL way to gain a six-pack from hell... Page 152

3 big reasons why—in prisons—leg raises have always been much more popular than sit-ups... Page 152

Why the hanging leg raise is the greatest single abdominal exercise known to man... Page 153

10 waist training secrets to help you master the hanging leg raise... Pages 154—155

How to correctly perform the greatest all-round midsection exercise in existence... Page 174

Going beyond the hanging straight leg raise... Page 178

Setting your sights on the most powerful midsection exercise possible—the V raise.... Page 178

How to develop abdominal muscles with enormous contractile power—and iron hip strength... Page 178

How to combat-proof your spine... Page 185

Why the bridge is the most important strength-building exercise in the world... Page 185

How to train your spine—as if your life depended on it... Page 185

Why you should sell your barbell set and buy a cushioned mat instead... Page 188

How to absorb punitive strikes against your spine—and bounce back smiling... Page 188

Why lower back pain is the foremost plague of athletes the world over... Page 189

Why bridging is the *ultimate* exercise for the spinal muscles... Page 189

The 4 signs of the perfect bridge... Page 191

How to master the bridge... Page 192

How to own a spine that feels like a steel whip... Page 193

How the bridging series will grant you an incredible combination of strength paired with flexibility... Page 216

Why bridging stands alone as a *total* training method that facilitates development in practically every area of fitness and health... Page 216

How to look exceptionally masculine—with broad, etched, and powerful shoulders... Page 219

Those vulnerable shoulders—why they ache and the best way to avoid or fix the pain... Page 220

How to choose authentic over *artificial* shoulder movements... Page 223

Why an understanding of *instinctive* human movement can help solve the shoulder pain problem... Page 224

Remove these two elements of pressing—and you will remove virtually all chronic shoulder problems... Page 225

The ultimate solution for safe, pain-free, powerful shoulders... Page 225

The mighty handstand pushup... Page 226

Using the handstand pushup to build *incredibly* powerful, muscularized shoulders in a short span of time... Page 225

How to strengthen the *vestibular system*—using handstand pushups... Page 225

8 secrets to help you perfect your all-important handstand pushup technique... Pages 228—229

Discover the ultimate shoulder and arm exercise... Page 248

Going beyond the one-arm handstand pushup... Page 252

The master of this old technique will have elbows strong as titanium axles... Page 255

The cast iron principles of Convict Conditioning success... Page 259

The missing "x factor" of training success... Page 259

The best ways to warm up... Page 260

How to create training momentum... Page 262

How to put strength in the bank... Page 263

This is the real way to get genuine, lasting strength and power gains... Page 265

Intensity—what it is and what it isn't... Page 265

Why "cycling" or "periodization" is unnecessary with bodyweight training... Page 266

How to make consistent progress... Page 266

5 powerful secrets for busting through your plateaus... Page 267

The nifty little secret of *consolidation* training... Page 268

Living by the buzzer—and the importance of regime... Page 275

5 major *Convict Conditioning* training programs... Page 276

The *New Blood* training program... Page 278

The *Good Behavior* training program... Page 279

The *Veterano* training program... Page 280

The *Solitary Confinement* training program... Page 281

The *Supermax* training program... Page 282

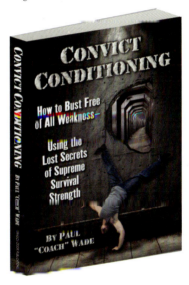

Convict Conditioning

How to Bust Free of All Weakness—Using the Lost Secrets of Supreme Survival Strength

By Paul "Coach" Wade

#B41 $39.95

Paperback 8.5 x 11   320 pages
191 photos, charts and illustrations

Dragon Door Customer Acclaim for Paul Wade's *Convict Conditioning*

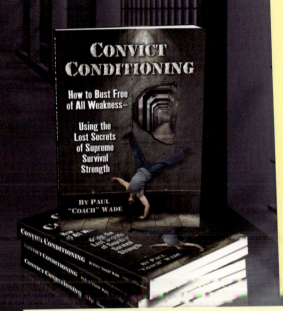

A Strength Training Guide That Will Never Be Duplicated!

"I knew within the first chapter of reading this book that I was in for something special and unique. The last time I felt this same feeling was when reading **Power to the People!** To me this is the Body Weight equivalent to Pavel's masterpiece.

Books like this can never be duplicated. Paul Wade went through a unique set of circumstances of doing time in prison with an 'old time' master of calisthenics. Paul took these lessons from this 70 year old strong man and mastered them over a period of 20 years while 'doing time'. He then taught these methods to countless prisoners and honed his teaching to perfection.

I believe that extreme circumstances like this are what it takes to create a true masterpiece. I know that 'masterpiece' is a strong word, but this is as close as it gets. No other body weight book I have read (and I have a huge fitness library)...comes close to this as far as gaining incredible strength from body weight exercise.

Just like Power to the People, I am sure I will read this over and over again...mastering the principles that Paul Wade took 20 years to master.

Outstanding Book!" —*Rusty Moore - Fitness Black Book* - Seattle, WA

A must for all martial artists

"As a dedicated martial artist for more than seven years, this book is exactly what I've been looking for.

For a while now I have trained with machines at my local gym to improve my muscle strength and power and get to the next level in my training. I always felt that the modern health club, technology based exercise jarred with my martial art though, which only required body movement.

Finally this book has come along. At last I can combine perfect body movement for martial skill with perfect body exercise for ultimate strength.

All fighting arts are based on body movement. This book is a complete textbook on how to max out your musclepower using only body movement, as different from dumbbells, machines or gadgets. For this reason it belongs on the bookshelf of every serious martial artist, male and female, young and old." —*Gino Cartier - Washington DC*

Brutal Elegance.

"I have been training and reading about training since I first joined the US Navy in the 1960s. I thought I'd seen everything the fitness world had to offer. Sometimes twice. But I was wrong. This book is utterly iconoclastic.

The author breaks down all conceivable body weight exercises into six basic movements, each designed to stimulate different vectors of the muscular system. These six are then elegantly and very intelligently broken into ten progressive techniques. You master one technique, and move on to the next.

The simplicity of this method belies a very powerful and complex training paradigm, reduced into an abstraction that obviously took many years of sweat and toil to develop.

Trust me. Nobody else worked this out. This approach is completely unique and fresh.

I have read virtually every calisthenics book printed in America over the last 40 years, and instruction like this can't be found anywhere, in any one of them. *Convict Conditioning* is head and shoulders above them all. In years to come, trainers and coaches will all be talking about 'progressions' and 'progressive calisthenics' and claim they've been doing it all along. But the truth is that Dragon Door bought it to you first. As with kettlebells, they were the trail blazers.

Who should purchase this volume? Everyone who craves fitness and strength should. Even if you don't plan to follow the routines, the book will make you think about your physical prowess, and will give even world class experts food for thought. At the very least if you find yourself on vacation or away on business without your barbells, this book will turn your hotel into a fully equipped gym.

I'd advise any athlete to obtain this work as soon as possible." —*Bill Oliver - Albany, NY, United States*

I've packed all of my other training books away!

"I read CC in one go. I couldn't put it down. I have purchased a lot of bodyweight training books in the past, and have always been pretty disappointed. They all seem to just have pictures of different exercises, and no plan whatsoever on how to implement them and progress with them. But not with this one. The information in this book is AWESOME! I like to have a clear, logical plan of progression to follow, and that is what this book gives. I have put all of my other training books away. CC is the only system I am going to follow. This is now my favorite training book ever!" —*Lyndan - Australia*

More Dragon Door Customer Acclaim for *Convict Conditioning*

Fascinating Reading and Real Strength

"Coach Wade's system is a real eye opener if you've been a lifetime iron junkie. Wanna find out how really strong (or weak) you are? Get this book and begin working through the 10 levels of the 6 power exercises. I was pleasantly surprised by my ability on a few of the exercises...but some are downright humbling. If I were on a desert island with only one book on strength and conditioning this would be it. (Could I staple Pavel's "Naked Warrior" to the back and count them as one???!) Thanks Dragon Door for this innovative new author." —**Jon Schultheis**, *RKC (2005) - Keansburg, NJ*

Single best strength training book ever!

"I just turned 50 this year and I have tried a little bit of everything over the years: martial arts, swimming, soccer, cycling, free weights, weight machines, even yoga and Pilates. I started using *Convict Conditioning* right after it came out. I started from the beginning, like Coach Wade says, doing mostly step one or two for five out of the six exercises. I work out 3 to 5 times a week, usually for 30 to 45 minutes.

Long story short, my weight went up 14 pounds (I was not trying to gain weight) but my body fat percentage dropped two percent. That translates into approximately 19 pounds of lean muscle gained in two months! I've never gotten this kind of results with anything else I've ever done. Now I have pretty much stopped lifting weights for strength training. Instead, I lift once a week as a test to see how much stronger I'm getting without weight training. There are a lot of great strength training books in the world (most of them published by Dragon Door), but if I had to choose just one, this is the single best strength training book ever. BUY THIS BOOK. FOLLOW THE PLAN. GET AS STRONG AS YOU WANT." —**Wayne** - *Decatur, GA*

Best bodyweight training book so far!

"I'm a martial artist and I've been training for years with a combination of weights and bodyweight training and had good results from both (but had the usual injuries from weight training). I prefer the bodyweight stuff though as it trains me to use my whole body as a unit, much more than weights do, and I notice the difference on the mat and in the ring. Since reading this book I have given the weights a break and focused purely on the bodyweight exercise progressions as described by 'Coach' Wade and my strength had increased more than ever before. So far I've built up to 12 strict one-leg squats each leg and 5 uneven pull ups each arm.

I've never achieved this kind of strength before - and this stuff builds solid muscle mass as well. It's very intense training. I am so confident in and happy with the results I'm getting that I've decided to train for a fitness/bodybuilding comp just using his techniques, no weights, just to show for real what kind of a physique these exercises can build. In sum, I cannot recommend 'Coach' Wade's book highly enough - it is by far the best of its kind ever!" —**Mark Robinson** - *Australia, currently living in South Korea*

A lifetime of lifting...and continued learning.

"I have been working out diligently since 1988 and played sports in high school and college before that. My stint the Army saw me doing calisthenics, running, conditioning courses, forced marches, etc. There are many levels of strength and fitness. I have been as big as 240 in my powerlifting/strongman days and as low as 185-190 while in the Army. I think I have tried everything under the sun: the high intensity of Arthur Jones and Dr. Ken, the Super Slow of El Darden, and the brutality of Dinosaur Training Brooks Kubic made famous.

This is one of the BEST books I've ever read on real strength training which also covers other just as important aspects of health; like staying injury free, feeling healthy and becoming flexible. It's an excellent book. He tells you the why and the how with his progressive plan. This book is a GOLD MINE and worth 100 times what I paid for it!"
—**Horst** - *Woburn, MA*

This book sets the standard, ladies and gentlemen

"It's difficult to describe just how much this book means to me. I've been training hard since I was in the RAF nearly ten years ago, and to say this book is a breakthrough is an understatement. How often do you really read something so new, so fresh? This book contains a complete new system of calisthenics drawn from American prison training methods. When I say 'system' I mean it. It's complete (rank beginner to expert), it's comprehensive (all the exercises and photos are here), it's graded (progressions from exercise to exercise are smooth and pre-determined) and it's totally original. Whether you love or hate the author, you have to listen to him. And you will learn something. This book just makes SENSE. In twenty years people will still be buying it." —**Andy McMann** - *Ponty, Wales, GB*

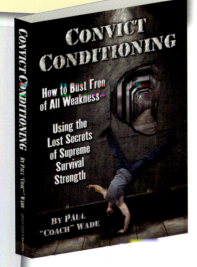

Convict Conditioning

How to Bust Free of All Weakness— Using the Lost Secrets of Supreme Survival Strength
By Paul "Coach" Wade

#B41 $39.95
Paperback 8.5 x 11 320 pages
191 photos, charts and illustrations

Advance Praise for Paul Wade's
Convict Conditioning 2

"Coach Paul Wade has outdone himself. His first book *Convict Conditioning* is to my mind THE BEST book ever written on bodyweight conditioning. Hands down. Now, with the sequel *Convict Conditioning 2*, Coach Wade takes us even deeper into the subtle nuances of training with the ultimate resistance tool: our bodies.

In plain English, but with an amazing understanding of anatomy, physiology, kinesiology and, go figure, psychology, Coach Wade explains very simply how to work the smaller but just as important areas of the body such as the hands and forearms, neck and calves and obliques in serious functional ways.

His minimalist approach to exercise belies the complexity of his system and the deep insight into exactly how the body works and the best way to get from A to Z in the shortest time possible.

I got the best advice on how to strengthen the hard-to-reach extensors of the hand right away from this exercise Master I have ever seen. It's so simple but so completely functional I can't believe no one else has thought of it yet. Just glad he figured it out for me.

Paul teaches us how to strengthen our bodies with the simplest of movements while at the same time balancing our structures in the same way: simple exercises that work the whole body.

And just as simply as he did with his first book. His novel approach to stretching and mobility training is brilliant and fresh as well as his take on recovery and healing from injury. Sprinkled throughout the entire book are too-many-to-count insights and advice from a man who has come to his knowledge the hard way and knows exactly of what he speaks.

This book is, as was his first, an amazing journey into the history of physical culture disguised as a book on calisthenics. But the thing that Coach Wade does better than any before him is his unbelievable progressions on EVERY EXERCISE and stretch! He breaks things down and tells us EXACTLY how to proceed to get to whatever level of strength and development we want. AND gives us the exact metrics we need to know when to go to the next level.

Adding in completely practical and immediately useful insights into nutrition and the mindset necessary to deal not only with training but with life, makes this book a classic that will stand the test of time.

Bravo Coach Wade, Bravo." —**Mark Reifkind, Master RKC,** author of *Mastering the Hardstyle Kettlebell Swing*

"The overriding principle of *Convict Conditioning 2* is 'little equipment-big rewards'. For the athlete in the throwing and fighting arts, the section on Lateral Chain Training, Capturing the Flag, is a unique and perhaps singular approach to training the obliques and the whole family of side muscles. This section stood out to me as ground breaking and well worth the time and energy by anyone to review and attempt to complete. Literally, this is a new approach to lateral chain training that is well beyond sidebends and suitcase deadlifts.

The author's review of passive stretching reflects the experience of many of us in the field. But, his solution might be the reason I am going to recommend this work for everyone: The Trifecta. This section covers what the author calls The Functional Triad and gives a series of simple progressions to three holds that promise to oil your joints. It's yoga for the strength athlete and supports the material one would find, for example, in Pavel's *Loaded Stretching*.

I didn't expect to like this book, but I come away from it practically insisting that everyone read it. It is a strongman book mixed with yoga mixed with street smarts. I wanted to hate it, but I love it."
—**Dan John,** author of *Don't Let Go* and co-author of *Easy Strength*

"I've been lifting weights for over 50 years and have trained in the martial arts since 1965. I've read voraciously on both subjects, and written dozens of magazine articles and many books on the subjects. This book and Wade's first, *Convict Conditioning*, are by far the most commonsense, information-packed, and result producing I've read. These books will truly change your life.

Paul Wade is a new and powerful voice in the strength and fitness arena, one that is commonsense, inspiring, and in your face. His approach to maximizing your body's potential is not the same old hackneyed material you find in every book and magazine piece that pictures steroid-bloated models screaming as they curl weights. Wade's stuff has been proven effective by hard men who don't tolerate fluff. It will work for you, too—guaranteed.

As an ex-cop, I've gone mano-y-mano with ex-cons that had clearly trained as Paul Wade suggests in his two *Convict Conditioning* books. While these guys didn't look like steroid-fueled bodybuilders (actually, there were a couple who did), all were incredibly lean, hard and powerful. Wade blows many commonly held beliefs about conditioning, strengthening, and eating out of the water and replaces them with result-producing information that won't cost you a dime." —**Loren W. Christensen,** author of *Fighting the Pain Resistant Attacker,* and many other titles

"*Convict Conditioning* is one of the most influential books I ever got my hands on. *Convict Conditioning 2* took my training and outlook on the power of bodyweight training to the 10th degree—from strengthening the smallest muscles in a maximal manner, all the way to using bodyweight training as a means of healing injuries that pile up from over 22 years of aggressive lifting.

I've used both *Convict Conditioning* and *Convict Conditioning 2* on myself and with my athletes. Without either of these books I can easily say that these boys would not be the BEASTS they are today. Without a doubt *Convict Conditioning 2* will blow you away and inspire and educate you to take bodyweight training to a whole NEW level."
—**Zach Even-Esh,** Underground Strength Coach

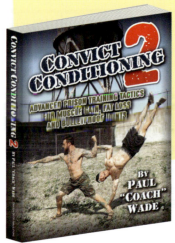

Convict Conditioning 2
Advanced Prison Training Tactics for Muscle Gain, Fat Loss and Bulletproof Joints
By Paul "Coach" Wade

#B59 $39.95
Paperback 8.5 x 11 354 pages
261 photos, charts and illustrations

 Mid-Level

 Advanced

Order *Convict Conditioning 2* online:
www.dragondoor.com/B59

24 HOURS A DAY ORDER NOW CALL 1•800•899•5111

*"Paul Wade's section on developing the sides of the body in **Convict Conditioning 2** is brilliant. Hardstyle!"* —**Pavel Tsatsouline**, author of *The Naked Warrior*

Online Praise for Convict Conditioning 2

Best Sequel Since The Godfather 2!
"Hands down the best addition to the material on *Convict Conditioning* that could possibly be put out. I already implemented the neck bridges, calf and hand training to my weekly schedule, and as soon as my handstand pushups and leg raises are fully loaded I'll start the flags. Thank you, Coach!"
— Daniel Runkel, Rio de Janeiro, Brazil

Just as brilliant as its predecessor!
"Just as brilliant as its predecessor! The new exercises add to the Big 6 in a keep-it-simple kind of way. Anyone who will put in the time with both of these masterpieces will be as strong as humanly possible. I especially liked the parts on grip work. To me, that alone was worth the price of the entire book."
—Timothy Stovall / Evansville, Indiana

Convict Conditioning 2
Advanced Prison Training Tactics for Muscle Gain, Fat Loss and Bulletproof Joints
By Paul "Coach" Wade

#B59 **$39.95**
Paperback 8.5 x 11   354 pages
261 photos, charts and illustrations

Mid-Level   Advanced

The progressions were again sublime
"Never have I heard such in depth and yet easy to understand description of training and physical culture. A perfect complement to the first book although it has its own style keeping the best attributes of style from the first but developing it to something unique. The progressions were again sublime and designed for people at all levels of ability. The two books together can forge what will closely resemble superhuman strength and an incredible physique and yet the steps to get there are so simple and easy to understand."
—Ryan O., Nottingham, United Kingdom

If you liked CC1, you'll love CC2
"*CC2* picks up where *CC1* left off with great information about the human flag (including a version called the clutch flag, that I can actually do now), neck and forearms. I couldn't be happier with this book."
—Justin B., Atlanta, Georgia

From the almost laughably-simple to realm-of-the-gods
"*Convict Conditioning 2* is a great companion piece to the original Convict Conditioning. It helps to further build up the athlete and does deliver on phenomenal improvement with minimal equipment and space.

The grip work is probably the superstar of the book. Second, maybe, is the attention devoted to the lateral muscles with the development of the clutch and press-flag.

Convict Conditioning 2 is more of the same - more of the systematic and methodical improvement in exercises that travel smoothly from the almost laughably-simple to realm-of-the-gods. It is a solid addition to any fitness library."
—Robert Aldrich, Chapel Hill, GA

Well worth the wait
"Another very interesting, and as before, opinionated book by Paul Wade. As I work through the CC1 progressions, I find it's paying off at a steady if unspectacular rate, which suits me just fine. No training injuries worth the name, convincing gains in strength. I expect the same with *CC2* which rounds off CC1 with just the kind of material I was looking for. Wade and Dragon Door deserve to be highly commended for publishing these techniques. A tremendous way to train outside of the gym ecosystem." —V. R., Bangalore, India

Very Informative
"*Convict Conditioning 2* is more subversive training information in the same style as its original. It's such a great complement to the original, but also solid enough on its own. The information in this book is fantastic-- a great buy! Follow this program, and you will get stronger."
—Chris B., Thunder Bay, Canada

Brilliant
"Convict Conditioning books are all the books you need in life. As Bruce Lee used to say, it's not a daily increase but a daily decrease. Same with life. Too many things can lead you down many paths, but to have Simplicity is perfect."—Brandon Lynch, London, England

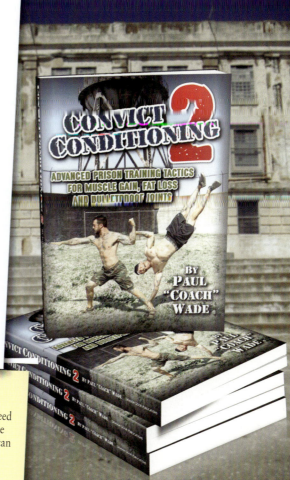

24 HOURS A DAY ORDER NOW CALL 1•800•899•5111

Order *Convict Conditioning 2* online:
www.dragondoor.com/B59

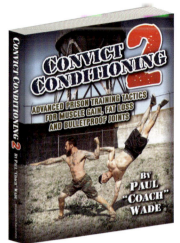

TABLE OF CONTENTS

Convict Conditioning 2
Advanced Prison Training Tactics for Muscle Gain, Fat Loss and Bulletproof Joints
By Paul "Coach" Wade

#B59 $39.95
Paperback 8.5 x 11   354 pages
261 photos, charts and illustrations

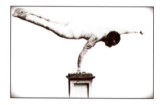

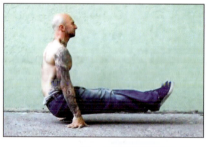

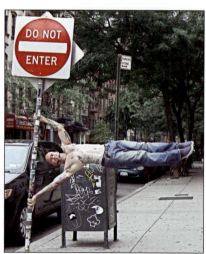

Foreword
The Many Roads to Strength by Brooks Kubik

Opening Salvo: *Chewing Bubblegum and Kicking Ass*

1. Introduction: *Put Yourself Behind Bars*

PART I: SHOTGUN MUSCLE

Hands and Forearms

2: Iron Hands and Forearms: *Ultimate Strength —with Just Two Techniques*

3: The Hang Progressions: *A Vice-Like Bodyweight Grip Course*

4: Advanced Grip Torture: *Explosive Power / Titanium Fingers*

5: Fingertip Pushups: *Keeping Hand Strength Balanced*

6: Forearms into Firearms: *Hand Strength: A Summary and a Challenge*

Lateral Chain

7: Lateral Chain Training: *Capturing the Flag*

8: The Clutch Flag: *In Eight Easy Steps*

9: The Press Flag: *In Eight Not-So-Easy Steps*

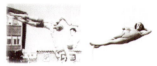

Neck and Calves

10. Bulldog Neck: *Bulletproof Your Weakest Link*

11. Calf Training: *Ultimate Lower Legs—No Machines Necessary*

PART II: BULLETPROOF JOINTS

12. Tension-Flexibility: *The Lost Art of Joint Training*

13. Stretching—the Prison Take: *Flexibility, Mobility, Control*

14. The Trifecta: *Your "Secret Weapon" for Mobilizing Stiff, Battle-Scarred Physiques—for Life*

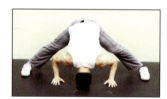

15: The Bridge Hold Progressions: *The Ultimate Prehab/Rehab Technique*

16: The L-Hold Progressions: *Cure Bad Hips and Low Back—Inside-Out*

17: Twist Progressions: *Unleash Your Functional Triad*

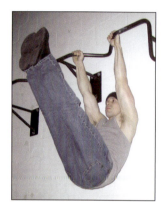

PART III: WISDOM FROM CELLBLOCK G

10. Doing Time Right: *Living the Straight Edge*

19. The Prison Diet: *Nutrition and Fat Loss Behind Bars*

20. Mendin' Up: *The 8 Laws of Healing*

21. The Mind: *Escaping the True Prison*

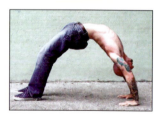

!BONUS CHAPTER!

Pumpin' Iron in Prison: *Myths, Muscle and Misconceptions*

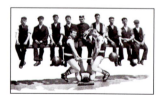

How to stay informed of the latest advances in strength and conditioning
Visit http://kbforum.dragondoor.com/

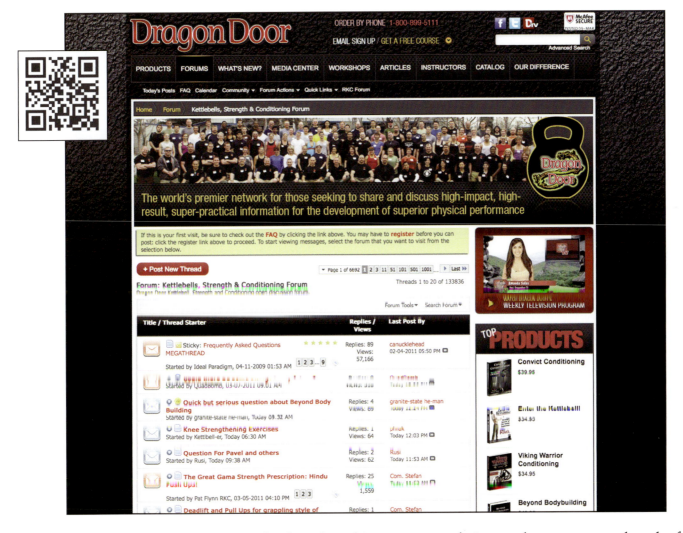

Visit www.dragondoor.com for late-breaking news and tips on how to stay ahead of the fitness pack.

Visit http://kbforum.dragondoor.com/ and participate in Dragon Door's stimulating and informative **Strength and Conditioning** Forum. Post your fitness questions or comments and get quick feedback from Pavel Tsatsouline and other leading fitness experts.

Visit www.dragondoor.com and browse the **Articles** section and other pages for groundbreaking theories and products for improving your health and well being.

24 HOURS A DAY ORDER NOW CALL 1·800·899·5111   www.dragondoor.com